HEALTH CARE IN TRANSITION

MEDICARE

FINANCING, INSOLVENCY AND FRAUD

HEALTH CARE IN TRANSITION

Additional books and e-books in this series can be found on Nova's website under the Series tab.

HEALTH CARE IN TRANSITION

MEDICARE

FINANCING, INSOLVENCY AND FRAUD

BRADFORD RODGERS
EDITOR

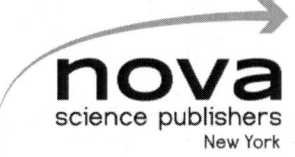

Copyright © 2019 by Nova Science Publishers, Inc.

All rights reserved. No part of this book may be reproduced, stored in a retrieval system or transmitted in any form or by any means: electronic, electrostatic, magnetic, tape, mechanical photocopying, recording or otherwise without the written permission of the Publisher.

We have partnered with Copyright Clearance Center to make it easy for you to obtain permissions to reuse content from this publication. Simply navigate to this publication's page on Nova's website and locate the "Get Permission" button below the title description. This button is linked directly to the title's permission page on copyright.com. Alternatively, you can visit copyright.com and search by title, ISBN, or ISSN.

For further questions about using the service on copyright.com, please contact:
Copyright Clearance Center
Phone: +1-(978) 750-8400   Fax: +1-(978) 750-4470   E-mail: info@copyright.com.

NOTICE TO THE READER

The Publisher has taken reasonable care in the preparation of this book, but makes no expressed or implied warranty of any kind and assumes no responsibility for any errors or omissions. No liability is assumed for incidental or consequential damages in connection with or arising out of information contained in this book. The Publisher shall not be liable for any special, consequential, or exemplary damages resulting, in whole or in part, from the readers' use of, or reliance upon, this material. Any parts of this book based on government reports are so indicated and copyright is claimed for those parts to the extent applicable to compilations of such works.

Independent verification should be sought for any data, advice or recommendations contained in this book. In addition, no responsibility is assumed by the publisher for any injury and/or damage to persons or property arising from any methods, products, instructions, ideas or otherwise contained in this publication.

This publication is designed to provide accurate and authoritative information with regard to the subject matter covered herein. It is sold with the clear understanding that the Publisher is not engaged in rendering legal or any other professional services. If legal or any other expert assistance is required, the services of a competent person should be sought. FROM A DECLARATION OF PARTICIPANTS JOINTLY ADOPTED BY A COMMITTEE OF THE AMERICAN BAR ASSOCIATION AND A COMMITTEE OF PUBLISHERS.

Additional color graphics may be available in the e-book version of this book.

Library of Congress Cataloging-in-Publication Data

ISBN: 978-1-53614-811-4

Published by Nova Science Publishers, Inc. † New York

CONTENTS

Preface vii

Chapter 1 Medicare: Insolvency Projections 1
Patricia A. Davis

Chapter 2 Medicare Financial Status: In Brief 17
Patricia A. Davis

Chapter 3 Medicare and Budget Sequestration 37
Ryan J. Rosso and Patricia A. Davis

Chapter 4 Medicare: CMS Should Take Actions to Continue Prior Authorization Efforts to Reduce Spending 65
United States Government Accountability Office

Chapter 5 Medicare: CMS Fraud Prevention System Uses Claims Analysis to Address Fraud 117
United States Government Accountability Office

Chapter 6 Medicare: Actions Needed to Better Manage Fraud Risks 145
Seto J. Bagdoyan

Index 177

PREFACE

Medicare is the nation's health insurance program for persons aged 65 and older and certain disabled persons. Medicare consists of four distinct parts: Part A (Hospital Insurance, or HI); Part B (Supplementary Medical Insurance, or SMI); Part C (Medicare Advantage, or MA); and Part D (the outpatient prescription drug benefit). Medicare covered over 58 million people in 2017 and has wide-ranging impact on the health-care sector and the overall U.S. economy. The Part A program is financed primarily through payroll taxes levied on current workers and their employers; these taxes are credited to the HI Trust Fund. From its inception, the HI Trust Fund has faced a projected shortfall. The 2018 Medicare Trustees Report projects that, under intermediate assumptions, the HI Trust Fund will become insolvent in 2026, three years earlier than estimated in the prior year's report as discussed in chapter 1. As reported in the next 2 chapters, spending under the program (except for a portion of administrative costs) is considered mandatory spending and is not subject to the appropriations process. Thus, there generally are no limits on annual Medicare spending. Medicare is most acutely impacted by the sequestration of mandatory funds, since Medicare benefit payments are considered mandatory spending. Special sequestration rules limit the extent to which Medicare can be reduced in a given fiscal year. Chapter 4 focuses on reducing expenditures, unnecessary utilization, and improper payments through prior authorization. The Centers for Medicare & Medicaid Services (CMS) has begun using prior authorization in Medicare through a series of fixed-length demonstrations designed to measure their effectiveness, and one permanent program. The billions of dollars in Medicare outlays as well as program complexity make it susceptible to improper payments, including fraud. Although there are no reliable estimates of fraud in Medicare, in fiscal year 2017 improper payments for Medicare were estimated at about $52 billion. The last 2 chapters address ways to prevent and manage Medicare fraud.

Chapter 1 - Medicare is the nation's health insurance program for persons aged 65 and older and certain disabled persons. Medicare consists of four distinct parts: Part A (Hospital Insurance, or HI); Part B (Supplementary Medical Insurance, or SMI); Part C (Medicare Advantage, or MA); and Part D (the outpatient prescription drug benefit).

The Part A program is financed primarily through payroll taxes levied on current workers and their employers; these taxes are credited to the HI Trust Fund. The Part B program is financed through a combination of monthly premiums paid by current enrollees and general revenues. Income from these sources is credited to the SMI Trust Fund. As an alternative, beneficiaries can choose to receive all their Medicare services through private health plans under the MA program; payment is made on beneficiaries' behalf in appropriate parts from the HI and SMI Trust Funds. The Part D drug benefit is funded through a separate account in the SMI Trust Fund and is financed through general revenues, state contributions, and beneficiary premiums. The HI and SMI Trust Funds are overseen by the Medicare Board of Trustees, which makes an annual report to Congress concerning the financial status of the funds.

From its inception, the HI Trust Fund has faced a projected shortfall. The insolvency date has been postponed a number of times, primarily due to legislative changes that have had the effect of restraining growth in program spending. The 2018 Medicare Trustees Report projects that, under intermediate assumptions, the HI Trust Fund will become insolvent in 2026, three years earlier than estimated in the prior year's report.

Preface

Chapter 2 - Medicare, administered by the Centers for Medicare and Medicaid Services (CMS), is the nation's federal insurance program that pays for covered health services for most persons aged 65 years and older and for most permanently disabled individuals under the age of 65. As a health insurance program, Medicare reimburses health care providers and suppliers, such as hospitals, physicians, and medical equipment companies, for the services and products they provide to Medicare beneficiaries. Medicare is prohibited by law from interfering in the practice of medicine or controlling the manner in which medical services are provided. It also is required to pay for covered services provided to eligible persons so long as specific criteria are met. As such, the growth in per person Medicare expenditures largely reflects the medical practices, use of technology, and underlying costs in the broader health care system. Spending under the program (except for a portion of administrative costs) is considered mandatory spending and is not subject to the appropriations process. Thus, there generally are no limits on annual Medicare spending.

Chapter 3 - Since its enactment in 1965, the Medicare program has undergone considerable change. Because of its rapid growth, both in terms of aggregate dollars and as a share of the federal budget, the Medicare program has been a major focus of deficit reduction legislation passed by Congress. With a few exceptions, reductions in program spending have been achieved largely through freezes or reductions in payments to providers, primarily hospitals and physicians, and by making changes to beneficiary premiums and other cost-sharing requirements. For example, the Patient Protection and Affordable Care Act (ACA; P.L. 111-148, as amended) made numerous changes to the Medicare program that modify provider reimbursements, provide incentives to improve the quality and efficiency of care, and enhance certain Medicare benefits.

Chapter 4 - CMS required prior authorization as a demonstration in 2012 for certain power mobility devices, such as power wheelchairs, in seven states. Under the prior authorization process, MACs review prior authorization requests and make determinations to approve or deny them based on Medicare coverage and payment rules. Approved requests will be paid as long as all other Medicare payment requirements are met.

GAO was asked to examine CMS's prior authorization programs. GAO examined 1) the changes in expenditures and the potential savings for items and services subject to prior authorization demonstrations, 2) reported benefits and challenges of prior authorization, and 3) CMS's monitoring of the programs and plans for future prior authorization. To do this, GAO examined prior authorization program data, CMS documentation, and federal internal control standards. GAO also interviewed CMS and MAC officials, as well as selected provider, supplier, and beneficiary groups.

Chapter 5 - CMS analyzes Medicare fee-forservice claims data to further its program integrity activities. In 2011, CMS implemented a data analytic system called FPS to develop leads for fraud investigations conducted by CMS program integrity contractors and to deny improper payments. In developing leads, FPS is intended to help CMS avoid improper payment costs by enabling quicker investigations and more timely corrective actions. Additionally, in 2012, CMS helped establish the HFPP to collaborate with other health care payers to address health care fraud. One of the key activities of the HFPP is to analyze claims data that are pooled from multiple payers, including private payers and Medicare.

GAO was asked to review CMS's use of FPS and the activities of the HFPP. This report examines 1) CMS's use of FPS to identify and investigate providers suspected of potential fraud, 2) the types of payments that have been denied by FPS, and 3) HFPP efforts to further CMS's and payers' ability to address health care fraud. GAO reviewed CMS documents, including reports to Congress on FPS, contractor statements of work, and information technology system user guides, and obtained fiscal year 2015 and 2016 data on FPS fraud investigations and claim denials. GAO also interviewed CMS officials and CMS program integrity contractors regarding how they use FPS, and a non-generalizable selection of HFPP participants regarding information and data sharing practices, and anti-fraud collaboration efforts.

Chapter 6 - Medicare covered over 58 million people in 2017 and has wide-ranging impact on the health-care sector and the overall U.S. economy. However, the billions of dollars in Medicare outlays as well as program complexity make it susceptible to improper payments, including fraud. Although there are no reliable estimates of fraud in Medicare, in fiscal year 2017 improper payments for Medicare were estimated at about $52 billion. Further, about $1.4 billion was returned to Medicare Trust Funds in fiscal year 2017 as a result of recoveries, fines, and asset forfeitures.

In December 2017, GAO issued a report examining how CMS managed its fraud risks overall and particularly the extent to which its efforts in the Medicare and Medicaid programs aligned with GAO's Framework. This testimony, based on that report, discusses the extent to which CMS's management of fraud risks in Medicare aligns with the Framework. For the report, GAO reviewed CMS policies and interviewed officials and external stakeholders.

In: Medicare: Financing, Insolvency and Fraud   ISBN: 978-1-53614-811-4
Editor: Bradford Rodgers   © 2019 Nova Science Publishers, Inc.

Chapter 1

MEDICARE: INSOLVENCY PROJECTIONS[*]

Patricia A. Davis

ABSTRACT

Medicare is the nation's health insurance program for persons aged 65 and older and certain disabled persons. Medicare consists of four distinct parts: Part A (Hospital Insurance, or HI); Part B (Supplementary Medical Insurance, or SMI); Part C (Medicare Advantage, or MA); and Part D (the outpatient prescription drug benefit).

The Part A program is financed primarily through payroll taxes levied on current workers and their employers; these taxes are credited to the HI Trust Fund. The Part B program is financed through a combination of monthly premiums paid by current enrollees and general revenues. Income from these sources is credited to the SMI Trust Fund. As an alternative, beneficiaries can choose to receive all their Medicare services through private health plans under the MA program; payment is made on beneficiaries' behalf in appropriate parts from the HI and SMI Trust Funds. The Part D drug benefit is funded through a separate account in the SMI Trust Fund and is financed through general revenues, state contributions, and beneficiary premiums. The HI and SMI Trust Funds

---

[*] This is an edited, reformatted and augmented version of Congressional Research Service, Publication No. RS20946, dated June 18, 2018.

are overseen by the Medicare Board of Trustees, which makes an annual report to Congress concerning the financial status of the funds.

From its inception, the HI Trust Fund has faced a projected shortfall. The insolvency date has been postponed a number of times, primarily due to legislative changes that have had the effect of restraining growth in program spending. The 2018 Medicare Trustees Report projects that, under intermediate assumptions, the HI Trust Fund will become insolvent in 2026, three years earlier than estimated in the prior year's report.

INTRODUCTION

Medicare is a federal insurance program that pays for covered health care services of qualified beneficiaries. It was established in 1965 under Title XVIII of the Social Security Act as a federal entitlement program to provide health insurance to individuals aged 65 and older, and it has been expanded over the years to include permanently disabled individuals under the age of 65.

Medicare consists of four distinct parts, A through D. Part A covers hospital services, skilled nursing facility (SNF) services, home health visits, and hospice services. Most persons aged 65 and older are automatically entitled to premium-free Part A because they or their spouse paid Medicare payroll taxes for at least 40 quarters (10 years) on earnings covered by either the Social Security or the Railroad Retirement systems. Part B covers a broad range of medical services, including physician services, laboratory services, durable medical equipment, and outpatient hospital services. Enrollment in Part B is voluntary; however, most beneficiaries with Part A also enroll in Part B. Part C, Medicare Advantage (MA), provides private plan options, such as managed care, for beneficiaries who are enrolled in both Part A and Part B. Part D provides optional outpatient prescription drug coverage.[1]

---

[1] For additional information on the Medicare program, see CRS Report R40425, *Medicare Primer*.

Medicare expenditures are driven by a variety of factors, including the level of enrollment, the complexity of medical services provided, health care inflation, and life expectancy. In 2017, Medicare provided benefits to about 58.4 million persons at an estimated total cost of $710.2 billion.[2]

The Medicare program has two separate trust funds—the Hospital Insurance (HI) Trust Fund and the Supplementary Medical Insurance (SMI) Trust Fund. The Part A program, which is financed mainly through payroll taxes levied on current workers, is accounted for through the HI Trust Fund. The Part B and Part D programs, which are funded primarily through general revenue and beneficiary premiums, are accounted for through the SMI Trust Fund.[3] Both funds are maintained by the Department of the Treasury and overseen by the Medicare Board of Trustees, which reports annually to Congress concerning the funds' financial status.[4] Financial projections are made using economic assumptions based on current law, including estimates of consumer price index, workforce size, wage increases, and life expectancy.

From its inception, the HI Trust Fund has faced a projected shortfall and eventual insolvency. Because of the way it is financed, the SMI Trust Fund cannot become insolvent; however, the Medicare trustees continue to express concerns about the rapid growth in SMI costs.[5]

MEDICARE HOSPITAL INSURANCE FINANCING

Similar to the Social Security system, the HI portion of Medicare was designed to be self-supporting and is financed through dedicated sources of

---

[2] Boards of Trustees, Federal Hospital Insurance and Federal Supplementary Medical Insurance Trust Funds, *2018 Annual Report of the Boards of Trustees of the Federal Hospital Insurance and Federal Supplementary Medical Insurance Trust Funds*, June 5, 2018, Table II.B, at https://www.cms.gov/Research-Statistics-Data-and-Systems/Statistics-Trends-and-Reports/ReportsTrustFunds/Downloads/TR2018.pdf.

[3] Payments are made for beneficiaries enrolled in Part C in appropriate portions from the Hospital Insurance (HI) and Supplementary Medical Insurance (SMI) Trust Funds.

[4] Medicare Trustees Reports may be found at http://www.cms.gov/Research-Statistics-Data-and-Systems/StatisticsTrends-and-Reports/ReportsTrustFunds/index.html.

[5] For further information on Medicare financing, see CRS Report R43122, *Medicare Financial Status: In Brief*.

income, rather than relying on general tax revenues. The primary source of income credited to the HI Trust Fund is *payroll taxes* paid by employees and employers; each pays a tax of 1.45% on earnings. The self-employed pay 2.9%. Unlike Social Security, there is no upper limit on earnings subject to the tax.[6] The Patient Protection and Affordable Care Act (ACA; P.L. 111-148, as amended) imposes an additional tax of 0.9% on high-income workers with wages over $200,000 for single filers and $250,000 for joint filers, effective for taxable years beginning in 2013.[7]

Additional income to the HI Trust Fund consists of premiums paid by voluntary enrollees who are not entitled to premium-free Medicare Part A through their (or their spouse's) work in covered employment, a portion of the federal income taxes paid on Social Security benefits,[8] and interest on federal securities held by the HI Trust Fund.

WHAT IS THE HI TRUST FUND?

The HI Trust Fund is a financial account in the U.S. Treasury into which all income to the Part A portion of the Medicare program is credited and from which all benefits and associated administrative costs of the Part A program are paid. The trust fund is solely an accounting mechanism—no actual money is transferred into or out of the fund.[9]

---

[6] Prior to 1991, the upper limit on taxable earnings was the same as for Social Security. The Omnibus Budget Reconciliation Act of 1990 (OBRA 90; P.L. 101-508) raised the limit in 1991 to $125,000. Under automatic indexing provisions, the maximum was increased to $130,200 in 1992 and $135,000 in 1993. The Omnibus Budget Reconciliation Act of 1993 (OBRA 93; P.L. 103-66) eliminated the upper limit entirely beginning in 1994.

[7] For additional detail, see archived CRS Report R41128, *Health-Related Revenue Provisions in the Patient Protection and Affordable Care Act (ACA)*.

[8] Since 1994, the HI Trust Fund has had an additional funding source; OBRA 93 increased the maximum amount of Social Security benefits subject to income tax from 50% to 85% and provided that the additional revenues would be credited to the HI Trust Fund.

[9] There are about 200 federal trust funds. For additional information on how federal trust funds operate within the context of the federal budget, see CRS Report R41328, *Federal Trust Funds and the Budget*.

HI operates on a "pay-as-you-go" basis, meaning the annual revenues to the HI Trust Fund, primarily the taxes paid by current workers and their employers, are used to pay Part A benefits for today's Medicare beneficiaries. When the government receives Medicare revenues (e.g., payroll taxes), income is credited by the Treasury to the appropriate trust fund in the form of special issue interest-bearing government securities.[10] (Interest on these securities is also credited to the trust fund.) The tax income exchanged for these securities then goes into the General Fund of the Treasury and is indistinguishable from other cash in the General Fund; this cash may be used for any government spending purpose. When payments for Medicare Part A services are made, the payments are paid out of the General Fund of the Treasury and a corresponding amount of securities is deleted from (written off) the HI Trust Fund.

In years in which the HI Trust Fund spends less than it receives in income, the fund has a *cash-flow surplus*. When this occurs, the HI Trust Fund securities exchanged for any income in excess of spending show up as assets on the trust fund's financial accounting balance sheets and are available to the system to meet future obligations. The trust fund surpluses are not reserved for future Medicare benefits but are simply bookkeeping entries that indicate how much Medicare has lent to the Treasury (or, alternatively, what is owed to Medicare by the Treasury). From a unified budget perspective, these assets represent future budget obligations and are treated as liabilities.[11]

If, in a given year, the HI Trust Fund spends more than it receives in income, the fund has a *cash-flow deficit*. In deficit years, Medicare can redeem any securities accumulated in previous years (including interest). When the securities are redeemed, the government needs to raise the resources necessary to pay for the securities and the monies are transferred

---

[10] Unlike marketable securities, special issues can be redeemed at any time at face value. Investment in special issues gives the trust funds the same flexibility as holding cash.

[11] For additional information, see Boards of Trustees, Federal Hospital Insurance and Federal Supplementary Medical Insurance Trust Funds, *The 2018 Annual Report of the Boards of Trustees of the Federal Hospital Insurance and Federal Supplementary Medical Insurance Trust Funds*, Appendix F, "Medicare and Social Security Trust Funds and the Federal Budget," June 5, 2018 at https://www.cms.gov/Research-Statistics-Data-and-Systems/Statistics-Trendsand-Reports/ReportsTrustFunds/Downloads/TR2018.pdf.

from the Treasury's General Fund to the HI Trust Fund. When the assets credited to the trust fund reach zero, the fund is deemed *insolvent*.

(See Appendix A for a discussion of recent and projected HI cash flows and for data on historical and projected HI operations through 2026).

HISTORY OF HI SOLVENCY PROJECTIONS

The HI Trust Fund has never become insolvent. The Medicare Board of Trustees projected insolvency for the HI Trust Fund beginning with the 1970 report,[12] at which time the trust fund was expected to become insolvent in only two years. (See Table 1 and Figure 1.) The insolvency date has been postponed a number of times since the beginning of Medicare through various methods. For example, the payroll tax rate has been adjusted periodically by Congress as one of the mechanisms to maintain the financial adequacy of the HI Trust Fund. (See Appendix B for historical payroll tax rates).

Other legislative changes have been made at various times to slow the growth in HI program spending; generally, these measures have been part of larger budget reconciliation laws that attempt to restrain overall federal spending. To illustrate, in the mid-1990s, efforts to curtail Medicare spending intensified as Congress considered legislation to bring the entire federal budget into balance and culminated in the passage of the Balanced Budget Act of 1997 (BBA 97; P.L. 105-33). In early 1997, the Medicare trustees had projected that the HI Trust Fund would become insolvent within four years, in 2001. Following the enactment of BBA 97, significant improvements were made in the short-term projections over the next few years. The new projections reflected a number of factors, including lower expected expenditures as a result of changes made by BBA 97 (primarily resulting from modifications in Medicare Part C payments and the

---

[12] Medicare Trustees Reports from 1966 through 1994 may be found on the Social Security History webpage at https://www.ssa.gov/history/reports/trust/trustyears.html. More recent reports may be found on the CMS webpage, "Trustees Report & Trust Funds," at https://www.cms.gov/Research-Statistics-Data-and-Systems/Statistics-Trendsand-Reports/ReportsTrustFunds/index.html.

establishment of prospective payment systems for certain Part A providers);[13] continued efforts to combat fraud and abuse; and strong economic growth, which was expected to generate more revenues to the trust fund from payroll taxes.

Table 1. Year of Projected Insolvency of the Hospital Insurance (HI) Trust Fund in Past and Current Trustees Reports

Year of Trustees Report	Year of Projected Insolvency	Year of Trustees Report	Year of Projected Insolvency	Year of Trustees Report	Year of Projected Insolvency
1970	1972	1986	1998 (amended)	2003	2026
1971	1973	1987	2002	2004	2019
1972	1976	1988	2005	2005	2020
1973	None Indicated	1989	None Indicated	2006	2018
1974	None Indicated	1990	2003	2007	2019
1975	Late 1990s	1991	2005	2008	2019
1976	Early 1990s	1992	2002	2009	2017
1977	Late 1980s	1993	1999	2010	2029
1978	1990	1994	2001	2011	2024
1979	1992	1995	2002	2012	2024
1980	1994	1996	2001	2013	2026
1981	1991	1997	2001	2014	2030
1982	1987	1998	2008	2015	2030
1983	1990	1999	2015	2016	2028
1984	1991	2000	2025	2017	2029
1985	1998	2001	2029	2018	2026
1986	1996	2002	2030	—	—

Sources: Intermediate projections of various Medicare Trustees Reports, 1970-2018.

---

[13] The Balanced Budget Act of 1997 (BBA 97; P.L. 105-33) established the Medicare + Choice program under Part C. Medicare Part C was changed to Medicare Advantage by the Medicare Prescription Drug, Improvement, and Modernization Act of 2003 (MMA; P.L. 108-173).

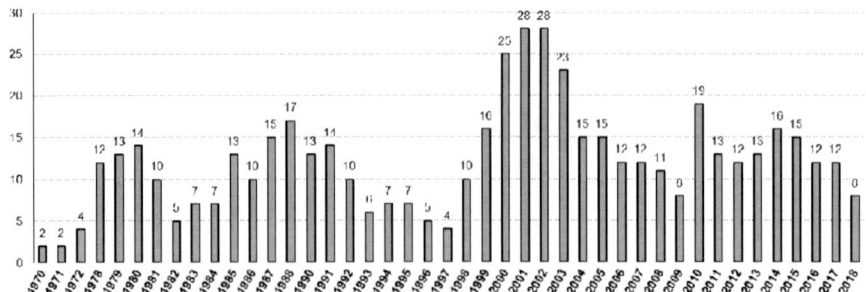

Sources: Intermediate projections of various Medicare Trustees Reports, 1970-2018.
Notes: No specific estimates were provided by the Medicare trustees for years 1973-1977 and 1989.

Figure 1. Projected Number of Years Until Medicare HI Trust Fund Insolvency.

There were concerns that the savings achieved through the enactment of BBA 97 were greater than intended at the time of enactment and had unintended consequences for health care providers. As a result of these concerns, Congress enacted two measures: the Balanced Budget Refinement Act of 1999 (BBRA 99; P.L. 106-113) and the Medicare, Medicaid, and SCHIP Benefits Improvement and Protection Act of 2000 (BIPA 2000; P.L. 106-554). These measures were designed to reverse some of the BBA 97 spending reductions.

Despite enactment of BBRA 99 and BIPA 2000, which increased program spending, the 2001 and 2002 Medicare Trustees Reports continued to delay the projected insolvency date. These improvements in solvency projections reflected both stronger-than-expected economic growth and lower-than-expected program costs due to lower projected enrollment in Medicare Part C, heightened antifraud and abuse initiatives, and lower-than-expected increases in health care costs.

The 2003 report projections, however, shifted direction. The projected insolvency date was 2026, four years earlier than the 2030 date projected in the 2002 report. The revision was due to lower-than-expected HI-taxable payroll and higher-than-expected hospital expenditures. In the next year, the 2004 report projected that the HI Trust Fund would become insolvent in 2019, seven years earlier than projected in 2003. A number of factors contributed to the revision of the projected insolvency date, including slow wage growth (on which payroll taxes are based) and faster growth in inpatient hospital benefits. In addition, the enactment of the Medicare Prescription Drug, Improvement, and Modernization Act of 2003 (MMA; P.L. 108-173) added significantly to HI costs, primarily through higher payments to rural hospitals and to private plans under the MA program.[14]

The 2005 Medicare Trustees Report projected that the HI Trust Fund would become insolvent one year later than projected in 2004, in 2020. The revision reflected slightly higher income and slightly lower costs in 2004 than previously estimated. The 2006 report moved the insolvency date forward again, to 2018. The revision reflected expectations of slightly higher costs and increased utilization of HI services. Both the 2007 and 2008 reports projected a 2019 insolvency date, although the 2008 report indicated that insolvency would occur earlier in the year. The 2009 report moved the insolvency date forward to 2017, due primarily to the economic recession.

The 2010 Medicare Trustees Report, issued subsequent to the enactment of the ACA, estimated that the combination of lower Part A costs and higher payroll-tax revenues expected to result from the ACA would postpone depletion of the HI Trust Fund's assets until 2029, 12 years later than the date projected in the 2009 report.[15] However, the 2011 report projected that the HI Trust Fund would become insolvent in 2024, five years earlier than projected in the 2010 report. The worsening financial outlook was primarily due to lowerthan-expected payroll taxes stemming from higher-than-expected unemployment and slow wage growth in 2010. The 2012 Medicare Trustees Report projected the same 2024 insolvency date. Although income from payroll taxes was expected to increase at a faster rate than expenditures through 2018 due to the projected economic recovery, the application of an additional 0.9% HI

---

[14] The Part D outpatient prescription drug program, which was created by the MMA, is funded under SMI; the increased expenditures associated with this new benefit therefore had little impact on projections of Medicare (HI) solvency.

[15] The expected reductions were primarily due to productivity adjustments to Part A provider payment updates and reduced payments to Medicare Advantage plans.

payroll tax for high-income workers beginning in 2013,[16] and the 2% reduction in spending required by the Budget Control Act of 2011 (BCA; P.L. 112-25) from 2013 through 2021,[17] income was still expected to be insufficient to fully cover projected HI expenses during that period.

In their 2013 report, the Medicare trustees projected a somewhat better short-term outlook for the HI Trust Fund. They moved the insolvency date two years later than their 2012 estimate, to 2026. The improved projections were primarily due to lower-than-expected expenditures in 2012, the base year used to project future expenditures, and a larger-than-estimated impact of ACA payment methodology changes on MA costs.[18] In their 2014 report, the Medicare trustees reported some improvement in Medicare's financial outlook and therefore moved the insolvency date four years later than their 2013 estimate, to 2030. This improvement was mainly due to lower expected utilization of and/or spending for certain Part A services, including inpatient hospital, skilled nursing, and home health care. The 2015 trustees report projected a similar short-term financial outlook and maintained the 2030 insolvency date estimate.

The 2016 Medicare Trustees Report projected a slightly worsened short-term outlook for the HI Trust Fund and therefore moved the insolvency date two years earlier than their 2015 estimate, to 2028. This change was primarily due to lower-than-expected payroll-tax income resulting from a slowing in real wage growth. In their 2017 report, the Medicare trustees projected a slightly improved short-term outlook for the HI Trust Fund and therefore moved the insolvency date one year later than their 2016 estimate, to 2029. This change was primarily due to lowerthan-expected HI expenditures in 2016 (which reduced the projection base) and lower projected future utilization of inpatient hospital services.

---

[16] The high-income payroll tax was added by the ACA. See "Medicare Hospital Insurance Financing."

[17] Subsequent legislation extended the reductions for an additional four years, through FY2025. For additional information on the Budget Control Act of 2011 (BCA; P.L. 112-25) and required Medicare spending reductions, see archived CRS Report R41965, *The Budget Control Act of 2011* and CRS Report R40425, *Medicare Primer*.

[18] See CRS Report R41196, *Medicare Provisions in the Patient Protection and Affordable Care Act (PPACA): Summary and Timeline*.

CURRENT INSOLVENCY PROJECTIONS

In their 2018 report,[19] the Medicare trustees projected a worsened short-term outlook for the HI Trust Fund and therefore moved the insolvency date three years earlier than their 2017 estimate, to 2026 (from 2029 in the 2017 report). This shift was primarily due to changes in estimates affecting HI revenues, including a reduction in projected income from payroll taxes due to lowerthan-expected wages in 2017 and projections of slower gross domestic product growth, as well as expectations of reduced income from taxes on Social Security benefits as a result of recent legislation that lowered individual income taxes through 2025.

While expenditures in the HI Trust Fund exceeded income each year from 2008 through 2015, the Medicare trustees reported small surpluses in 2016 and 2017. (See Table A-1.) In 2018 and beyond, however, expenditure growth is expected to again outpace growth in income. Trust fund assets would be used to make up the difference between income and expenditures, until the assets were depleted in 2026. (See Figure 2).

Each year, beginning in 2010, the Centers for Medicare & Medicaid Services (CMS) actuaries have issued an illustrative alternative scenario that has assumed that certain ACA changes that reduce Part A provider reimbursements would be gradually phased out.[20] As the 2018 alternative scenario assumes that this phaseout would begin in 2028, after the projected 2026 HI insolvency date, this alternative analysis assumes the same 2026 date of insolvency.

---

[19] Boards of Trustees, Federal Hospital Insurance and Federal Supplementary Medical Insurance Trust Funds, *2018 Annual Report of the Boards of Trustees of the Federal Hospital Insurance and Federal Supplementary Medical Insurance Trust Funds*, June 5, 2018, at https://www.cms.gov/Research-Statistics-Data-and-Systems/Statistics-Trendsand-Reports/ReportsTrustFunds/Downloads/TR2018.pdf.

[20] Memo from John D. Shatto and M. Kent Clemens, "Projected Medicare Expenditures under an Illustrative Scenario with Alternative Payment Updates to Medicare Providers," June 5, 2018, at https://www.cms.gov/Research-StatisticsData-and-Systems/Statistics-Trends-and-Reports/ReportsTrustFunds/Downloads/2018TRAlternativeScenario.pdf.

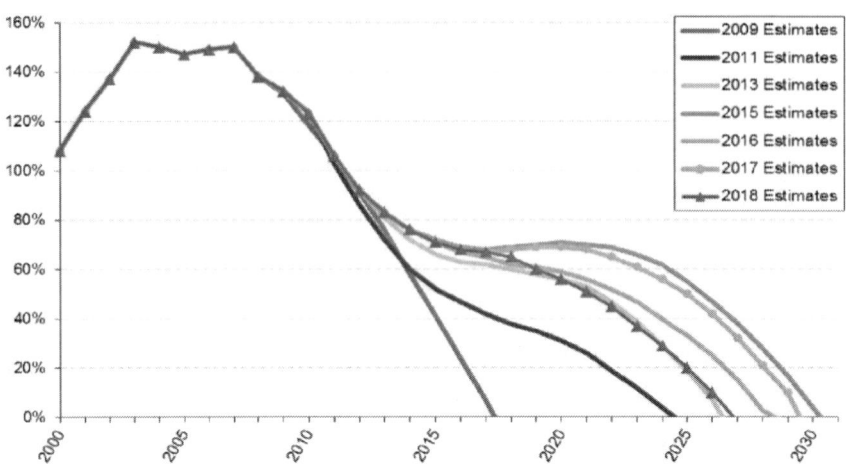

Sources: Data from the Boards of Trustees, Federal Hospital Insurance and Federal Supplementary Medical Insurance Trust Funds, 2009 Annual Report of the Boards of Trustees of the Federal Hospital Insurance and the Federal Supplementary Medical Insurance Trust Funds, Table II.E1, and Summaries of the 2011 through 2017 Annual Reports of the Social Security and Medicare Boards of Trustees, Chart D (2011) and Chart E (2013, 2015, 2016, 2017, and 2018).

Notes: The 2010 estimated insolvency date was 2029. The 2012 insolvency date estimate was the same as the date projected in the 2011 report (2024), and the 2014 insolvency date estimate was the same as that in the 2015 report (2030).

Figure 2. HI Trust Fund Assets at Beginning of Year as a Percentage of Annual Expenditures; (estimates from selected 2009-2018 Medicare Trustees Reports).

WHAT WOULD HAPPEN IF THE FUND BECAME INSOLVENT?

The practical function of the HI Trust Fund is to permit the continued payment of bills in the event of a temporary financial strain (e.g., lower income or higher costs than expected) without requiring legislative action. As long as the HI Trust Fund has a balance (i.e., securities are credited to the fund), the Treasury Department is authorized to make payments for Medicare Part A services. If the HI Trust Fund is not able to pay all current expenses out of current income and accumulated trust fund assets, the HI Trust Fund is considered to be *insolvent*.[21]

To date, the HI Trust Fund has never become insolvent. There are no provisions in the Social Security Act that govern what would happen if insolvency were to occur. For example, the program has no statutory authority to use general revenues to fund Part A services in the event of such a shortfall.

In their 2018 report, the Medicare trustees project that the HI Trust Fund will be exhausted in 2026. At that time, HI would continue to receive tax income from which some benefits could be paid; however, funds would be sufficient to pay for only 91% of Part A expenses. Unless action is taken prior to that date to increase revenues or to decrease expenditures (or some combination of the two), Congress may face a legislative decision regarding whether, and how, to provide for another source of funding (e.g., general revenues) to make up for these deficits.

MEDICARE FINANCING ISSUES

Much of the concern about the financial status of Medicare tends to focus on the HI Trust Fund date of insolvency, when Medicare no longer has the authority to pay for Part A health care services in full. This focus can, however, detract from the larger issues confronting the Medicare program as a whole and from the program's current and future impact on the federal budget and on taxpayers. When viewed from the perspective of the entire federal budget, as the number of beneficiaries and per capita health care costs continue to grow, total Medicare spending obligations (HI

---

[21] From time to time, it is reported that Medicare is on the verge of "bankruptcy"; however, in the context of federal trust funds, this term is not meaningful. It is true that a trust fund's outgo can be greater than its income and that trust funds can have a zero balance, but, unlike private businesses, the federal government is not in danger of "going out of business" or having its assets seized by creditors. As noted, Congress has often taken actions to increase the trust fund's revenues or reduce its outgo when the Medicare HI Trust Fund has faced imminent insolvency.

and SMI spending combined) are expected to place increasing demands on federal budgetary resources.

As noted earlier, because of the way it is financed, the SMI (Parts B and D) portion of Medicare cannot become insolvent. However, a continuing shift from providing care in inpatient (Part A) settings to outpatient (Parts B and D) settings has resulted in a greater portion of Medicare spending being covered by beneficiary premiums and general revenues than by dedicated payroll taxes.[22] In the future, the Medicare trustees estimate that the portion of personal and corporate income taxes needed to fund SMI will increase from about 15.4% in 2017 to about 22.0% in 2030 and 26.3% in 2092.[23]

APPENDIX A. OPERATION OF THE HOSPITAL INSURANCE TRUST FUND

Beginning in 2004, expenditures began exceeding *tax* income (from payroll taxes and from the taxation of Social Security benefits). Expenditures began to exceed *total* income (tax income plus all other sources of revenue) in 2008, and Hospital Insurance (HI) assets (the balance of the HI Trust Fund at the beginning of the year) were used to meet the portion of expenditures that exceeded income. Expenditures exceeded income every year from 2008 through 2015. In 2016 and 2017, the HI Trust Fund ran a small surplus. Beginning in 2018, expenditures are expected to again exceed income each year, with trust fund assets making up the difference, until the asset balance is depleted in 2026. At that time, the HI Trust Fund would no longer have sufficient funds to allow for the full payment of Part A expenditures (see Table A-1, below, for historical and projected Medicare financial data through 2027).

---

[22] The Congressional Budget Office estimated that the share of Medicare spending financed by dedicated payroll taxes declined from 67% in 2000 to about 39% in 2016. Congressional Budget Office, *The 2016 Long-Term Budget Outlook*, July 2016, p. 44, at https://www.cbo.gov/publication/51580.

[23] This amount is separate from and in addition to the payroll taxes used to fund the Part A (HI) portion of the program.

Table A-1. Operation of the Hospital Insurance Trust Fund, Calendar Years 1970-2027 (in billions of dollars)

Year	Income			Expenditures			Trust Fund	
	Payroll Taxes	Interest, Transfers, Other[a]	Total	Benefit Payments	Admin. Expenses	Total	Net Change from Prior Year	Balance at End of Year
Historical Data								
1970	$4.9	$1.2	$6.0	$5.1	$0.2	$5.3	$0.7	$3.2
1975	11.5	1.4	13.0	11.3	0.3	11.6	1.4	10.5
1980	23.8	2.1	26.1	25.1	0.5	25.6	0.5	13.7
1985	47.6	3.9	51.4	47.6	0.8	48.4	4.8	20.5
1990	72.0	8.4	80.4	66.2	0.8	67.0	13.4	98.9
1995	98.4	16.7	115.0	116.4	1.2	117.6	-2.6	130.3
2000	144.4	22.9	167.2	128.5	2.6	131.1	36.1	177.5
2005	171.4	28.0	199.4	180.0	2.9	182.9	16.4	285.8
2006	181.3	30.2	211.5	189.0	2.9	191.9	19.6	305.4
2007	191.9	31.9	223.7	200.2	2.9	203.1	20.7	326.0
2008	198.7	32.0	230.8	232.3	3.3	235.6	-4.7	321.3
2009	190.9	34.5	225.4	239.3	3.2	242.5	-17.1	304.2
2010	182.0	33.7	215.6	244.5	3.5	247.9	−32.3	271.9
2011	195.6	33.4	228.9	252.9	3.8	256.7	−27.7	244.2
2012	205.7	37.3	243.0	262.9	3.9	266.8	−23.8	220.4
2013	220.8	30.3	251.1	261.9	4.3	266.2	−15.0	205.4
2014	227.4	33.9	261.2	264.9	4.5	269.3	−8.1	197.3
2015	241.1	34.3	275.4	273.4	5.5	278.9	−3.5	193.8
2016	253.5	37.3	290.8	280.5	4.9	285.4	5.4	199.1
2017	261.5	37.8	299.4	293.3	3.2	296.5	2.8	202.0
Intermediate Estimates								
2018	268.0	37.5	305.5	305.5	5.2	310.7	−5.2	196.8
2019	286.5	38.5	325.0	322.7	5.5	328.2	−3.1	193.6
2020	302.0	41.4	343.4	342.6	5.9	348.5	−5.1	188.5
2021	318.3	44.3	362.7	366.4	6.3	372.7	−10.1	178.4
2022	335.2	47	382.3	393.9	6.8	400.7	−18.4	160.0
2023	352.6	49.7	402.3	422.6	7.2	429.8	−27.5	132.6
2024	370.9	52.7	423.5	451.9	7.7	459.5	−36.1	96.5
2025	389.1	55.8	444.8	482.6	8.2	490.8	−46.0	50.5
2026	408.1	62.6	470.8	514.0	8.7	522.7	−51.9	−1.4
2027	426.8	70.6	497.5	545.5	9.4	554.8	−57.3	−58.7

Source: Boards of Trustees, Federal Hospital Insurance and Federal Supplementary Medical Insurance Trust Funds, 2018 Annual Report of the Boards of Trustees of the Federal Hospital Insurance and Federal Supplementary Medical Insurance Trust Funds, June 5, 2018, Table III.B4.

Notes: Sums may not equal totals due to rounding.

[a] Includes income from the taxation of Social Security benefits, Railroad Retirement account transfers, premiums paid by voluntary enrollees, and interest.

APPENDIX B. HISTORICAL PAYROLL TAX RATES

Table B-1. Tax Rates and Maximum Tax Bases

Calendar Year	Maximum Tax Base	Tax Rate (percentage of taxable earnings)	
		Employees and Employers, Each	Self-Employed
1966	$6,600	0.35%	0.35%
1967	6,600	0.50	0.50
1968-1971	7,800	0.60	0.60
1972	9,000	0.60	0.60
1973	10,800	1.00	1.00
1974	13,200	0.90	0.90
1975	14,100	0.90	0.90
1976	15,300	0.90	0.90
1977	16,500	0.90	0.90
1978	17,700	1.00	1.00
1979	22,900	1.05	1.05
1980	25,900	1.05	1.05
1981	29,700	1.30	1.30
1982	32,400	1.30	1.30
1983	35,700	1.30	1.30
1984	37,800	1.30	2.60
1985	39,600	1.35	2.70
1986	42,000	1.45	2.90
1987	43,800	1.45	2.90
1988	45,000	1.45	2.90
1989	48,000	1.45	2.90
1990	51,300	1.45	2.90
1991	125,000	1.45	2.90
1992	130,200	1.45	2.90
1993	135,000	1.45	2.90
1994-2012	no limit	1.45	2.90
2013 and later[a]	no limit	1.45	2.90

Source: 2018 Medicare Trustees Report, Table III.B2.

[a] Beginning in 2013, workers pay an additional 0.9% of their earnings above $200,000 (those who file individual tax returns) or $250,000 (those who file joint tax returns).

In: Medicare: Financing, Insolvency and Fraud ISBN: 978-1-53614-811-4
Editor: Bradford Rodgers © 2019 Nova Science Publishers, Inc.

Chapter 2

MEDICARE FINANCIAL STATUS: IN BRIEF[*]

Patricia A. Davis

OVERVIEW OF THE MEDICARE PROGRAM

Medicare, administered by the Centers for Medicare and Medicaid Services (CMS), is the nation's federal insurance program that pays for covered health services for most persons aged 65 years and older and for most permanently disabled individuals under the age of 65.[1] As a health insurance program, Medicare reimburses health care providers and suppliers, such as hospitals, physicians, and medical equipment companies, for the services and products they provide to Medicare beneficiaries. Medicare is prohibited by law from interfering in the practice of medicine or controlling the manner in which medical services are provided. It also is required to pay for covered services provided to eligible persons so long as specific criteria are met. As such, the growth in per person Medicare

---

[*] This is an edited, reformatted and augmented version of Congressional Research Service, Publication No. R43122, dated July 2, 2018.

[1] For additional information on the Medicare program, see CRS Report R40425, *Medicare Primer*.

expenditures largely reflects the medical practices, use of technology, and underlying costs in the broader health care system. Spending under the program (except for a portion of administrative costs) is considered mandatory spending and is not subject to the appropriations process. Thus, there generally are no limits on annual Medicare spending.

Since its enactment in 1965, the Medicare program has undergone considerable change. Because of its rapid growth, both in terms of aggregate dollars and as a share of the federal budget, the Medicare program has been a major focus of deficit reduction legislation passed by Congress.[2] With a few exceptions, reductions in program spending have been achieved largely through freezes or reductions in payments to providers, primarily hospitals and physicians, and by making changes to beneficiary premiums and other cost-sharing requirements. For example, the Patient Protection and Affordable Care Act (ACA; P.L. 111-148, as amended) made numerous changes to the Medicare program that modify provider reimbursements, provide incentives to improve the quality and efficiency of care, and enhance certain Medicare benefits.[3]

Four Parts of Medicare

Medicare consists of four distinct parts, A through D:

- Part A covers inpatient hospital services, skilled nursing care, hospice care, and some home health services. Most persons aged 65 and older are automatically entitled to premium-free Part A because they or their spouse paid Medicare payroll taxes for at

---

[2] For a brief history of changes to the Medicare program, see CRS Report R40425, *Medicare Primer*, and the Medicare chapter of the House of Representatives, Committee on Ways and Means, *Greenbook,* at http://greenbook.waysandmeans.house.gov/2016-green-book/chapter-2-medicare.

[3] For details on individual Medicare provisions in the Patient Protection and Affordable Care Act (ACA; 111-148, as amended), see CRS Report R41196, *Medicare Provisions in the Patient Protection and Affordable Care Act (PPACA): Summary and Timeline*.

least 40 quarters (10 years) on earnings covered by either the Social Security or the Railroad Retirement systems.
- Part B covers a broad range of medical services, including physician services, laboratory services, durable medical equipment, and outpatient hospital services. Enrollment in Part B is optional; however, most beneficiaries with Part A also enroll in Part B.
- Part C (Medicare Advantage, or MA) is a private plan option for beneficiaries that covers all Parts A and B services, except hospice. Individuals choosing to enroll in Part C must be eligible for Part A and also must enroll in Part B. About one-third of Medicare beneficiaries are enrolled in MA.[4]
- Part D covers outpatient prescription drug benefits. This portion of the program is optional. About 76% of Medicare beneficiaries are enrolled in Medicare Part D or have coverage through an employer retiree plan subsidized by Medicare.[5]

Beneficiary Costs

In addition to paying premiums for Medicare Parts B and D,[6] beneficiaries must pay other out-of-pocket costs, such as deductibles and coinsurance, for services provided under all parts of the Medicare program. There is no limit on beneficiary out-of-pocket spending, and most beneficiaries have some form of supplemental insurance through private Medigap plans, employer-sponsored retiree plans, or Medicaid to help cover a portion of their Medicare premiums and/or deductibles and coinsurance.

---

[4] Boards of Trustees of the Federal Hospital Insurance and Federal Supplementary Medical Insurance Trust Funds, The 2018 Annual Report of the Boards of Trustees of the Federal Hospital Insurance and Federal Supplementary Medical Insurance Trust Funds, June 5, 2018, Table V.B3.

[5] Ibid.

[6] Beneficiaries enrolled in a Medicare Advantage (MA; Part C) plan must pay Part B premiums as well as any additional premium required by the MA plan.

Provider and Plan Payments

Under traditional Medicare, Parts A and B, the government generally pays providers directly for services on a *fee-for-service* basis using different prospective payment systems, or fee schedules.[7] Under Parts C and D, Medicare pays private insurers a monthly *capitated* per person amount to provide coverage to enrollees. The capitated payments are adjusted to reflect differences in the relative cost of sicker beneficiaries with different risk factors including age, disability, or end-stage renal disease.

MEDICARE TRUST FUNDS AND SOURCES OF REVENUE

The Medicare program has two separate trust funds—the Hospital Insurance (HI) Trust Fund for Part A and the Supplementary Medical Insurance (SMI) Trust Fund for Parts B and D.[8] (For beneficiaries enrolled in MA [Part C], payments are made on their behalf in appropriate portions from the HI and SMI Trust Funds.) Both the HI and SMI Trust Funds are maintained by the Department of the Treasury and overseen by a Medicare Board of Trustees that reports annually to Congress concerning the funds'

---

[7] Under a *prospective payment system* (PPS), Medicare payments are made using a predetermined, fixed amount based on the classification system for a particular service. The Centers for Medicare & Medicaid Services (CMS) uses separate PPSs to reimburse acute inpatient hospitals, home health agencies, hospice, hospital outpatient departments, inpatient psychiatric facilities, inpatient rehabilitation facilities, long-term care hospitals, and skilled nursing facilities. A *fee schedule* is a listing of fees used by Medicare to pay doctors or other providers/suppliers. Fee schedules are used to pay for physician services; ambulance services; clinical laboratory services; and durable medical equipment, prosthetics, orthotics, and supplies in certain locations.

[8] Many government programs are financed through trust funds. Despite the name, federal trust funds are not the same as private-sector trust funds. A trust in the private sector is a fiduciary relationship in which one person (the trustee) holds property for the benefit of another (the beneficiary). The trustee must follow the express terms of the trust instrument and administer the trust for the benefit of the beneficiary. Most federal trust funds are not based on a legal fiduciary relationship. Congress creates trust funds that involve a commitment to use monies for a specific purpose, but it can alter the terms (e.g., receipts, outlays, or purpose) of the trust fund at any time. For additional information, see CRS Report R41328, *Federal Trust Funds and the Budget*.

financial status.⁹ Financial projections are made using economic assumptions based on current law, including estimates of consumer price index (CPI), workforce size, wage increases, and life expectancy.

The Medicare trust funds are financial accounts in the U.S. Treasury into which all income to the program is credited and from which all benefits and associated administrative costs of the program are paid. The trust funds are solely accounting mechanisms—there is no actual transfer of money into and out of the funds. As long as a trust fund has a balance, the Department of the Treasury is authorized to make payments for it from the U.S. Treasury.

Hospital Insurance Trust Fund

The Part A portion of Medicare is financed through the HI Trust Fund.

Sources of HI Revenue

The HI Trust Fund is funded primarily by a dedicated payroll tax of 2.9% of earnings, shared equally between employers and workers. (See *Figure 1*.) Unlike Social Security, there is no upper limit on wages subject to Medicare payroll taxes. Beginning in 2013, the ACA has imposed an additional tax of 0.9% on high-income workers with wages over $200,000 for single tax filers and over $250,000 for joint filers.[10] Other sources of income to the HI Trust Fund include premiums paid by voluntary enrollees who are not entitled to premium-free Medicare Part A, a portion of the federal income taxes paid on Social Security benefits, and interest on federal securities held by the trust fund.

---

[9] These reports may be found at https://www.cms.gov/Research-Statistics-Data-and-Systems/Statistics-Trends-andReports/ReportsTrustFunds/index.html.

[10] See CRS Report R41128, *Health-Related Revenue Provisions in the Patient Protection and Affordable Care Act (ACA)*, for more detail.

HI Trust Fund Mechanics

HI operates on a pay-as-you-go basis; the taxes paid by current workers and their employers are used to pay Part A benefits for today's Medicare beneficiaries. When the government receives Medicare revenues (payroll taxes), income is credited by the Treasury to the HI Trust Fund in the form of special-issue interest-bearing government securities.[11] (Interest on these securities also is credited to the trust fund.) The tax income exchanged for these securities then goes into the general fund of the Treasury and is indistinguishable from other cash in the general fund; this cash may be used for any government spending purpose. When payments for Medicare Part A services are made, the payments are paid out of the general treasury and a corresponding amount of securities is deleted from (written off) the HI Trust Fund.

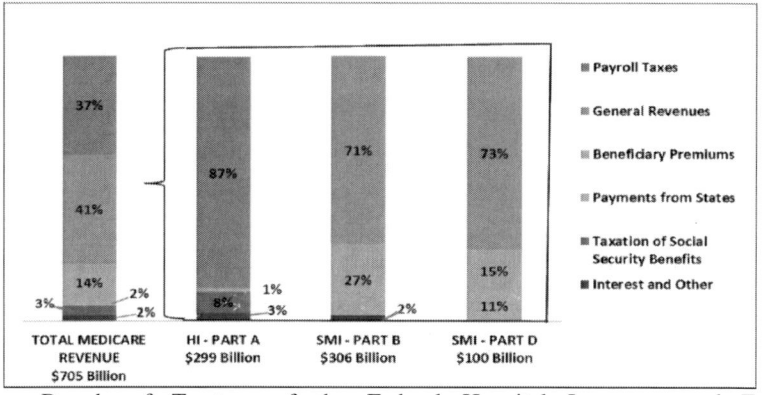

Source: Boards of Trustees of the Federal Hospital Insurance and Federal Supplementary Medical Insurance Trust Funds, The 2018 Annual Report of the Boards of Trustees of the Federal Hospital Insurance and Federal Supplementary Medical Insurance Trust Funds, June 5, 2018, Table II.B1.

Notes: Totals may not add to 100% due to rounding. HI = Hospital Insurance; SMI = Supplementary Medical Insurance. In 2017, Part B premiums represented over 25% of Part B income due, in part, to a $3.00 per month Part B premium surcharge imposed by the Bipartisan Budget Act of 2015 (P.L. 114-74).

Figure 1. Sources of Medicare Revenues: 2017.

---

[11] Unlike marketable securities, special issues can be redeemed at any time at face value. Investment in special issues gives the trust funds the same flexibility as holding cash.

In years in which the trust fund spends less than the income it receives, the trust fund securities exchanged for any income in excess of spending show up as *assets* on the financial accounting balance sheets and are available to the system to meet future obligations. The trust fund surpluses are not reserved for future Medicare benefits but are simply bookkeeping entries that indicate how much Medicare has lent to the Treasury (or alternatively, what is owed to Medicare by the Treasury). From a unified budget perspective, these assets represent future budget obligations and are treated as liabilities. If the HI Trust Fund is not able to pay all current expenses out of current income and accumulated trust fund assets, it is considered to be *insolvent*.[12]

Supplementary Medical Insurance Trust Fund

The SMI Trust Fund consists of two accounts: Part B and Part D.

Sources of SMI Revenue

Unlike the HI portion of Medicare, the SMI program was not intended to be supported through dedicated sources of income. Instead, it relies primarily on general tax revenues and beneficiary premiums as revenue sources.[13]

The Part B portion of SMI is funded mainly through beneficiary premiums (set at 25% of estimated program costs for the aged)[14] and general revenues (most of the remaining amount, approximately 75%). In

---

[12] From time to time, it is reported that Medicare is on the verge of *bankruptcy*; however, in the context of federal trust funds, this term is not meaningful. Although a federal trust fund's spending can be greater than its income and trust funds can have a zero balance, unlike private businesses, the federal government is not in danger of "going out of business" or having its assets seized by creditors.

[13] There have been reports that Medicare beneficiaries receive more from the program than what they have paid throughout their working years in payroll taxes; however, as noted, unlike Part A, the costs of Medicare Parts B and D were designed in the original statute to be subsidized by the government and not through dedicated taxes.

[14] For additional information, see CRS Report R40082, *Medicare: Part B Premiums*.

2018, the standard monthly Part B premium is $134.00.[15] However, certain low-income enrollees receive assistance with their premiums from Medicaid (joint federal-state funding), and, since 2007, high-income enrollees pay higher premiums. Beginning in 2011, additional revenues from an annual fee imposed on certain manufacturers and importers of branded prescription drugs also are credited to the SMI Trust Fund.[16]

Part D is financed through a combination of beneficiary premiums (set at 25.5% of the estimated cost of the standard benefit), general revenues, and state transfer payments (to cover a portion of the costs of beneficiaries enrolled in both Medicare and Medicaid—the *dual-eligibles*). Actual Part D premiums may vary depending on which plan the enrollee selects. Low-income enrollees may receive premium assistance through the Part D low-income subsidy (all federal funding), and, starting in 2011, higher income enrollees pay higher premiums.

SMI Trust Fund Mechanics

The level of SMI funding is automatically updated each year to cover expenditures in the upcoming year. If actual costs exceed those estimated when the funding was set, the amount of financing in the next year (i.e., general revenues and beneficiary premiums) may be adjusted to recover the shortfall. Similarly, if actual costs are less than expected in a given year, income levels needed for the next year may be adjusted downward. Because of these automatic adjustments, the SMI Trust Fund is always kept in balance and cannot become insolvent.

---

[15] However, in 2018, about 28% of Part B enrollees are protected by a provision in the Social Security Act (the *hold-harmless provision*) that prevents their Medicare premiums from increasing more than the annual increase in their Social Security benefit payments. These individuals pay less than $134 per month in 2018. For additional information, see CRS Report R40082, *Medicare: Part B Premiums*.

[16] This revenue source is included in "Interest and Other" for Part B in *Figure 1*. For additional detail, see CRS Report R41128, *Health-Related Revenue Provisions in the Patient Protection and Affordable Care Act (ACA)*.

MEDICARE SPENDING IN 2017[17]

In calendar year (CY) 2017, Medicare provided benefits to about 58.4 million people (49.5 million people aged 65 and older and 8.9 million disabled people under the age of 65) at an estimated total cost of $710 billion.[18] Most of that amount, about $702 billion (99%), was spent on program benefits, with the remaining amount used for program administration. (See *Table 1*.)

Table 1. Medicare Expenditures and Enrollment: CY2017

	HI	SMI		
	Part A	Part B	Part D	Total
Expenditures (billions)				
Benefits	$293.3	$308.6	$100.1	$702.1
Hospital	144.6	53.3	—	197.9
Skilled Nursing	28.3	—	—	28.3
Home Health Care	6.9	11.5	—	18.4
Physician Services	—	69.1	—	69.1
Private Plans (Part C)	94.5	115.1	—	209.7
Prescription Drugs	—	—	100.1	100.1
Other	19.1	59.6	—	78.8
Administrative Expenses	3.2	5.0	−0.1	$8.1
Total Expenditures	$296.5	$313.7	$100.0	$710.2
Enrollment (millions)				
Aged	49.2	45.3	37.3	49.5
Disabled	8.9	8.1	7.1	8.9
Total Enrollment	58.0	53.4	44.5	58.4
Average expenditures per enrollee	$5,055	$5,780	$2,252	$13,087

Source: 2018 Report of the Medicare Trustees, Table II.B1.
Notes: Totals do not necessarily equal the sums of rounded components.

---

[17] Data is from the Boards of Trustees of the Federal Hospital Insurance and Federal Supplementary Medical Insurance Trust Funds, *The 2018 Annual Report of the Boards of Trustees of the Federal Hospital Insurance and Federal Supplementary Medical Insurance Trust Funds*, June 5, 2018 (hereinafter, the 2018 Report of the Medicare Trustees).

[18] This amount reflects Medicare total spending regardless of revenue source; it does not net out nonfederal income (e.g., premiums, state transfers). By law, the Medicare Trustees Report focuses on the financial status of the program's trust funds and does not examine the impact of Medicare spending on the overall federal budget.

2017 HI Operations

At the beginning of CY2017, the HI Trust Fund had an asset balance of about $199 billion. During 2017, Part A expenditures were about $297 billion. Approximately $262 billion of that amount was funded by payroll taxes and $38 billion by interest income and other sources. (See "Sources of HI Revenue.") Because revenue income exceeded expenditures, about $3 billion in surplus accumulated in the HI Trust Fund. At the end of 2017, the HI Trust Fund had an asset balance of approximately $202 billion. This means that if or when HI spending exceeds income in future years, the trust fund will be able to spend a total of $202 billion in addition to what it receives in income.[19]

2017 SMI Operations

In CY2017, total spending for Part B was close to $314 billion, with general revenues financing approximately $217 billion of that amount and premiums covering most of the remainder. Total spending for Part D reached about $100 billion in 2017, with more than $73 billion of that amount paid for by general revenues. In addition, approximately $11 billion was covered by state transfer payments, and $16 billion was covered by beneficiary premiums. It should be noted that although beneficiary premiums are set at a rate to cover 25.5% of the costs of standard Part D benefits, the program pays for the premiums of about one-third of enrollees because these enrollees qualify for low-income assistance. As a result, Part D premiums represented about 15% of Part D revenues in 2017. (See *Figure 1.*)

---

[19] In years in which income exceeds expenditures, the surplus amount(s) would be added to this balance.

ESTIMATED DATE OF HI TRUST FUND INSOLVENCY

From 2008 to 2015, Part A expenditures exceeded HI income each year, and the assets credited to the trust fund were drawn down to make up the deficit. In 2016 and 2017, the HI Trust Fund ran a small surplus;[20] however, the Medicare trustees project a return to deficits in 2018 and in the following years until the HI Trust Fund becomes depleted (insolvent) in 2026. At that time, there would no longer be sufficient funds to fully cover Part A expenditures; although HI would continue to receive tax income, the funds would cover only 91% of Part A expenses. The trustees suggest that, under these circumstances, beneficiary access to Part A services "could rapidly be curtailed."[21]

Almost from its inception, the HI Trust Fund has faced a projected shortfall and eventual insolvency (see *Figure 2*), with insolvency dates ranging from 2 years to 28 years from the year of the projection. However, to date, the HI Trust Fund has never become insolvent. There are no provisions in the Social Security Act that govern what would happen if that were to occur; for example, there is no authority in law for the program to use general revenues to fund Part A services in the event of such a shortfall. Unless action is taken prior to the expected date of insolvency to increase HI revenues or decrease expenditures, Congress may face a decision regarding the provision of additional funding to make up for these deficits and to allow for full and on-time payments to Part A providers.

Because income (general revenue and premiums) to the SMI Trust Fund is updated automatically each year to ensure that the program has enough money to continue operating, the SMI Trust Fund is kept in balance and is always solvent. However, the Medicare trustees continue to express concerns about the rapid growth in SMI (Parts B and D) costs.

---

[20] The trustees attributed this period of surplus to low spending growth for Part A services, to a strengthening economy, and to the continued sequestration of 2% of Medicare benefit spending.

[21] The 2018 Report of the Medicare Trustees, p. 26.

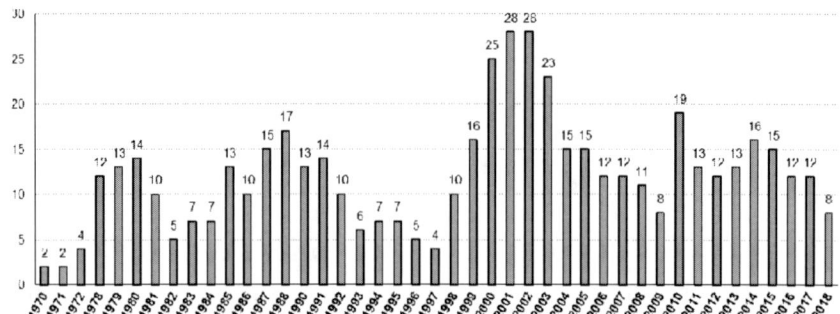

Source: Intermediate projections of various Medicare Trustees Reports, 1970-2018.
Notes: No specific estimates were provided by the trustees for years 1973-1977 and 1989.

Figure 2. Projected Number of Years Until Hospital Insurance Insolvency.

PROJECTED MEDICARE SPENDING GROWTH

Although the 2018 Medicare Trustees Report notes a recent slowing in the growth of U.S. national health expenditures,[22] the trustees still project that U.S. health care expenditures, including Medicare spending, will grow faster than gross domestic product (GDP) in most future years. For Medicare, the projected growth in the prices of health services plus anticipated increases in utilization rates and in the complexity of services provided are expected to contribute to rising costs of Medicare relative to GDP. The aging of the baby boom population is also expected to contribute to significant increases in benefit expenditures.[23]

Over the next 10 years, the Medicare trustees estimate that total Medicare expenditures will increase from $710 billion in 2017 to close to $1.44 trillion in 2027. Of the $1.44 trillion, about $555 billion is expected

---

[22] The trustees are uncertain whether this slowing is of limited duration (e.g., due to recent economic downturns) or whether it may be a longer-term trend due to structural changes in the health care industry.

[23] When Medicare first began, there were about 19 million beneficiaries. This number has grown to almost 60 million enrollees in 2018 and is expected to increase to about 80 million in 2030 and close to 118 million in 2092.

to be spent on Part A services, $685 billion on Part B services, and $195 billion on Part D services. (See *Figure 3*.)

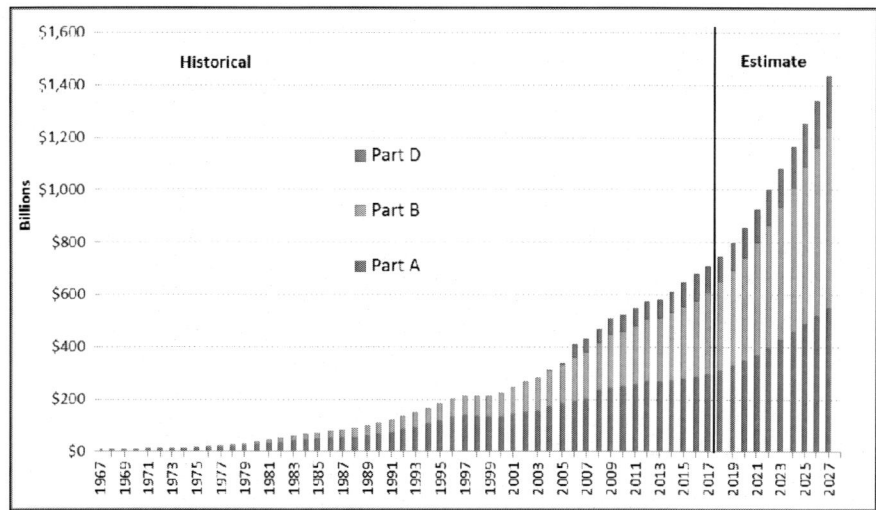

Source: 2018 Report of the Medicare Trustees, Expanded and Supplementary Tables (historical data); and Report Tables III.B4; III.C4; and III.D3 (projected data).

Figure 3. Historical and Projected Medicare Expenditures.

Growth in Medicare Expenditures Relative to GDP

A comparison of Medicare expenditures (for Medicare Parts A through D, combined) to GDP provides a measure of the amount of financial resources that will be necessary to pay for Medicare services relative to the output of the U.S. economy. Under current law, the trustees expect total Medicare expenditures to increase from 3.7% of GDP in 2018 to about 5.9% of GDP by 2042, mainly due to the rapid growth in the number of beneficiaries, and then to about 6.2% of GDP in 2092, with growth in health care cost per beneficiary becoming the more significant factor in those years. (See *Figure 4*.)

Over the next 75 years, general revenues and beneficiary premiums are expected to play an increasing role in financing the program. For example, the level of general revenues needed to fund SMI is expected to increase from 1.6% of GDP in 2018 to an estimated 2.8% in 2092 under current law.[24] Similarly, income from beneficiary premiums is expected to increase from 0.6% of GDP in 2018 to 1.0% in 2092. In 2017, about 15.4% of total federal income taxes collected that year were used to fund the general revenue portion of SMI. It is expected that the portion of personal and corporate income taxes needed to fund SMI will increase to about 22% in 2030 and to about 26% in 2092. This amount is *in addition to* the payroll taxes used to fund the Part A (HI) portion of the program.

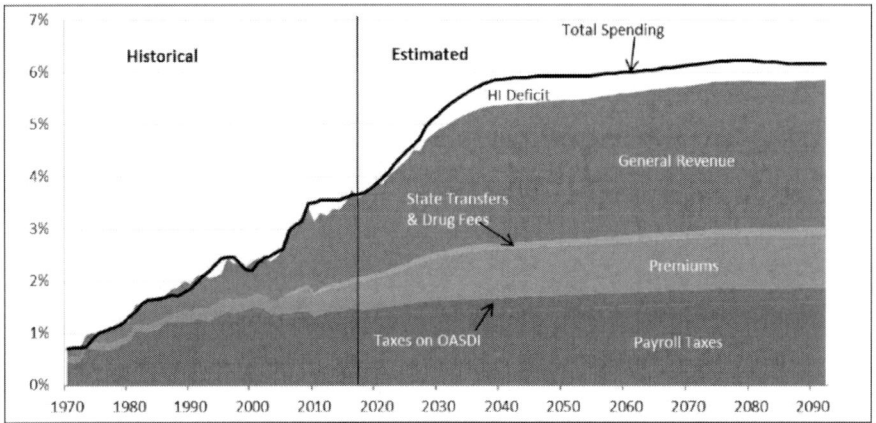

Source: Summary of the 2018 Annual Reports of the Social Security and Medicare Boards of Trustees, Chart C, at http://www.ssa.gov/oact/TRSUM/index.html.

Figure 4. Medicare Cost and Non-interest Income, by Source as a Percentage of GDP.

Unfunded and General Revenue Obligations

The trustees report provides estimates of the present value of the HI deficit—the *unfunded obligation*—over both a 75-year horizon and an "infinite" horizon. (See *Table 2*.) This unfunded obligation represents the dollar amount by which expenditures would need to be reduced or revenue increased to maintain the financial soundness of the program over a period

---

[24] Total Part B outlays were over 1.6% of GDP in 2017, and the trustees project that they will grow to close to 2.8% of GDP by 2092. The trustees also estimate that total Part D outlays will increase from about 0.5% of GDP in 2017 to over 1.2% of GDP in 2092.

of time. The trustees estimate that the current value of funding needed to cover the expected difference between income to the HI Trust Fund and expenditures over the next 75 years is $4.5 trillion. The trustees note that this financial imbalance could be addressed by immediately increasing payroll taxes to 3.72% (from the current 2.9%), or by immediately decreasing expenditures by 17%, or by some combination of the two. From a budgetary standpoint, the accumulated assets in the trust fund are considered liabilities, as the redemption of the assets represents a formal budget commitment. Therefore, the starting balance of $0.2 trillion in the HI Trust Fund needs to be added to the unfunded obligation of $4.5 trillion for a present value of $4.7 trillion shortfall in dedicated revenues.

The trustees report also provides estimates of the present value of future SMI spending. Although SMI is funded automatically and does not face a shortfall, the general revenue portion represents obligated federal spending. The present value of expected general revenues needed to pay for Medicare Parts B and D over the next 75 years is $33.0 trillion. Adding the HI unfunded obligation estimate and the present value of future SMI spending for the 75-year period yields a total of $37.7 trillion.[25] In other words, it would take about $37.7 trillion in current dollars to cover the cost of Medicare not funded through dedicated sources over the next 75 years.

Comparison to Prior-Year Estimates

Over both the short and long terms, projections of total Medicare spending in the 2018 trustees report are higher than those in the 2017 report. (See *Figure 5*.)

---

[25] The trustees note that while SMI general revenue transfers represent formal budget commitments under current law, no provision exists for covering the NI Trust Fund once assets are depleted.

Table 2. Current Value of Estimated Medicare Unfunded Obligations and General Revenue Spending

Present Value of HI Deficit		Present Value of SMI General Revenues			
	Part A		Part B	Part D	Total
Unfunded obligations through 2092	$4.7 trillion[a]	General revenue contributions through 2092	$25.1 trillion	$7.9 trillion	$37.7 trillion
Unfunded obligations through infinite horizon	-$2.0 trillion[a]	General revenue contributions through infinite horizon	$46.4 trillion	$19.3 trillion	$63.7 trillion

Source: 2018 Report of the Medicare Trustees, Tables V.F2, V.G1, V.G3, V.G5.

[a]. Budgetary and trust fund accounting rules differ in the treatment of trust fund assets. From a budgetary standpoint, the accumulated assets in the trust fund are considered liabilities, as the redemption of the assets represents a formal budget commitment. The starting balance of $0.2 trillion in the HI Trust Fund is thus included in this figure. Under trust fund accounting methods, which exclude the asset balance, the unfunded HI obligation for the 75-year projection period would be $4.5 trillion and -$2.2 trillion for the infinite projection period.

Both the short-term and the long-term financial outlooks for the HI Trust Fund have somewhat deteriorated compared to estimates in last year's report. The estimated depletion date of the HI Trust Fund is 2026, three years earlier than projected in the 2017 report. Over the next 75 years, the estimated HI actuarial deficit (the amount that would need to be added to the payroll tax to maintain HI solvency for this period) increased by 0.18%—from 0.64% of taxable payroll in the 2017 report to 0.82% of taxable payroll in the 2018 report. This increase is due to expected changes in both HI income and costs. The increase in projected HI costs is primarily due to higher-than-expected Part A expenditures in 2017 (which increases the projection base), recent legislation that increased hospital spending, and higher Medicare Advantage payments. The projected decrease in income is due to expected reductions in payroll taxes as a result of lower than expected wages in 2017 and lower projected GDP, and to expected reductions in income from the taxation of Social Security benefits as a result of recent tax legislation.

Part B projected short- and long-term costs are also higher in the 2018 report due to higher Medicare Advantage spending and recent legislation that ended caps for certain therapy services and eliminated the Independent Payment Advisory Board.[26] In the short term, projected Part D costs are slightly lower than estimates in last year's report due to an expected increase in manufacturer rebates provided to Part D plans, and a decline in spending for hepatitis C and diabetes drugs. However, due to an assumption of a slightly higher growth rate in Part D, long-range projections of Part D spending remain similar to the trustees' 2017 projections.

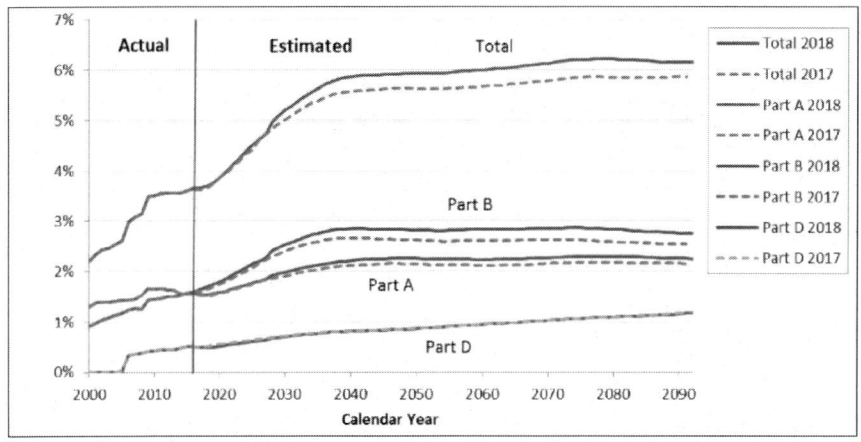

Sources: 2017 and 2018 Medicare Trustees Reports, Supplementary Tables.

Figure 5. Comparison of 2017 and 2018 Medicare Expenditure Projections. (expenditures as a percentage of GDP)

Alternative Projections

Throughout the 2018 report, the Medicare trustees caution that actual costs may be higher than their intermediate projections. For example,

---

[26] See CRS Report R45126, Bipartisan Budget Act of 2018 (P.L. 115-123): Brief Summary of Division E—The Advancing Chronic Care, Extenders, and Social Services (ACCESS) Act.

because the trustees are required to base their estimates on current law, their assumptions assume that physician payments will be updated according to levels set forth in the Medicare Access and CHIP Reauthorization Act of 2015 (MACRA; P.L. 114-10),[27] and that the full ACA-required Medicare plan and provider payment reductions will be maintained.

Because of concerns about the accuracy of these projections, the Medicare trustees asked the CMS Office of the Actuary to prepare an alternative projection based on the assumptions that annual physician payment updates will transition beginning in 2028 from current law to 2.2% by 2042, that the 5% bonuses for physicians in the advanced alternative payment models (APM) and the $500 million in additional payments to physicians in the merit-based incentive system (MIPS) will continue after 2025, and that ACA provider payment adjustments will be phased down beginning in 2028.[28] Under this alternative scenario, long-term Medicare costs are projected to reach about 8.9% of GDP in 2092, instead of 6.2% under the trustees' current-law projections. Additionally, under the alternative scenario, the HI actuarial deficit would be 1.71% of taxable payroll (compared with 0.82% under the current-law projection), which could be addressed by immediately increasing payroll taxes to 4.61% or by immediately decreasing expenditures by 30% (compared with 3.72% and 17%, respectively, under current law). Because the differences in assumptions between current law and the alternative scenario do not begin until 2028, the alternative scenario projects the same 2026 date of HI insolvency.

---

[27] See CRS Report R43962, The Medicare Access and CHIP Reauthorization Act of 2015 (MACRA; P.L. 114-10).

[28] John D. Shatto and M. Kent Clemens, "Projected Medicare Expenditures under an Illustrative Scenario with Alternative Payment Updates to Medicare Providers," June 5, 2018, at https://www.cms.gov/Research-Statistics-Dataand-Systems/Statistics-Trends-and-Reports/ReportsTrustFunds/Downloads/2018TRAlternativeScenario.pdf.

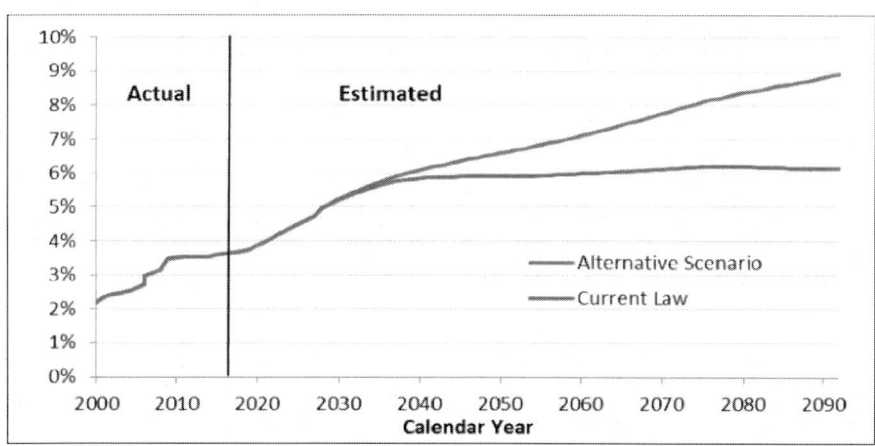

Source: 2018 Report of the Medicare Trustees, Supplementary Tables.

Note: The alternative scenario assumes phasing out certain MACRA and ACA provider payment reductions.

Figure 6. Comparison of Medicare Expenditure Projections Based on Current Law and an Alternative Scenario. (expenditures as a percentage of GDP)

In: Medicare: Financing, Insolvency and Fraud ISBN: 978-1-53614-811-4
Editor: Bradford Rodgers © 2019 Nova Science Publishers, Inc.

Chapter 3

MEDICARE AND BUDGET SEQUESTRATION[*]

Ryan J. Rosso and Patricia A. Davis

ABSTRACT

Sequestration is the automatic reduction (i.e., cancellation) of certain federal spending, generally by a uniform percentage. The sequester is a budget enforcement tool that was established by Congress in the Balanced Budget and Emergency Deficit Control Act of 1985 (BBEDCA; also known as the Gramm-Rudman-Hollings Act; P.L. 99-177) and was intended to encourage compromise and action, rather than actually being implemented (also known as "triggered"). Generally, this budget enforcement tool has been incorporated into laws to either discourage Congress from violating specific budget objectives or encourage Congress to fulfill specific budget objectives. When Congress breaks these types of rules, either through the enactment of a law or lack thereof, a sequester is triggered and certain federal spending is reduced.

Sequestration is of recent interest due to its current use as an enforcement mechanism for three budget enforcement rules created by the Statutory Pay-As-You-Go Act of 2010 (Statutory PAYGO, P.L. 111-139) and the Budget Control Act of 2011 (BCA, P.L. 112-25). Currently, only the BCA mandatory sequester is triggered, resulting in the

---

[*] This is an edited, reformatted and augmented version of Congressional Research Service, Publication No. R45106, dated February 16, 2018.

sequestration of mandatory funds through FY2027. However, the Statutory PAYGO sequester and BCA discretionary sequester are current law and can be triggered if associated budget enforcement rules are broken.

Medicare is a federal program that pays for certain health care services of qualified beneficiaries. The program is funded using both mandatory and discretionary spending and is impacted by any sequestration order issued in accordance with the aforementioned laws. Medicare is most acutely impacted by the sequestration of mandatory funds, since Medicare benefit payments are considered mandatory spending. Special sequestration rules limit the extent to which Medicare can be reduced in a given fiscal year. Most notably, rules cap the percentage reduction that can be applied to Medicare's benefit payments, but this sequestration cap varies depending on the type of sequestration order.

Under a BCA mandatory sequestration order, Medicare benefit payments and Medicare Integrity Program spending cannot be reduced by more than 2%. Under a Statutory PAYGO sequestration order, Medicare benefit payments and Medicare Program Integrity spending cannot be reduced by more than 4%. These limits do not apply to mandatory administrative Medicare spending under either type of sequestration order. These limits also do not apply to discretionary administrative Medicare spending under a BCA discretionary sequestration order.

Generally, Medicare's benefit structure remains unchanged under a mandatory sequestration order, and beneficiaries see few direct impacts. However, due to varying financing structures between the four parts of the program, sequestration has been implemented differently across the program.

INTRODUCTION

Sequestration is the automatic reduction (i.e., cancellation) of certain federal spending, generally by a uniform percentage.[1] The sequester is a budget enforcement tool that Congress established in the Balanced Budget and Emergency Deficit Control Act of 1985 (BBEDCA; also known as the

---

[1] Under the Balanced Budget and Emergency Deficit Control Act of 1985 (BBEDCA; also known as the GrammRudman-Hollings Act; P.L. 99-177) Sec. 250(c)(2), sequestration is defined as "the cancellation of budgetary resources provided by discretionary appropriations or direct spending law." Budgetary resources are subject to sequestration unless exempted by law. See OMB Circular A-11, Section 100. https://www.whitehouse.gov/sites/whitehouse.gov/files/omb/assets/a11_current_year/a11_2017/s100.pdf.

Gramm-Rudman-Hollings Act; P.L. 99-177) intended to encourage compromise and action, rather than actually being implemented (also known as "triggered").[2] Generally, this budget enforcement tool has been incorporated into laws to either discourage Congress from violating specific budget objectives or encourage Congress to fulfill specific budget objectives. When Congress breaks these types of rules, either through the enactment of a law or lack thereof, a sequester is triggered and certain federal spending is reduced.

Sequestration is of recent interest due to its current use as an enforcement mechanism for three budget enforcement rules created by the Statutory Pay-As-You-Go Act of 2010 (Statutory PAYGO, P.L. 111-139) and the Budget Control Act of 2011 (BCA, P.L. 112-25). Currently, only the BCA mandatory sequester is triggered, but the Statutory PAYGO sequester and BCA discretionary sequester are current law and can be triggered if the budget enforcement rules are broken.

Medicare,[3] which is a federal program that pays for covered health care services of qualified beneficiaries, is subject to a reduction in federal spending associated with the implementation of these three sequesters, although special rules limit the extent to which it is impacted.

This report begins with an overview of budget sequestration and Medicare before discussing how budget sequestration has been implemented across the different parts of the Medicare program. Additionally, this chapter provides an appendix of budget terminology definitions, as defined by BBEDCA.

BUDGET SEQUESTRATION

Under current law, sequestration is a budget enforcement tool that occurs because certain policy goals have not been met. When a sequester is triggered, all applicable budget accounts, unless exempted by law, are

---

[2] U.S. Congress, Senate Committee on Finance, *Budget Enforcement Mechanisms*, Oral and Written Testimony of the Honorable Phil Gramm, 112th Cong., 1st sess., May 4, 2011.
[3] For more information on Medicare, see CRS Report R40425, *Medicare Primer*, coordinated by Patricia A. Davis.

reduced by a percentage amount for a fiscal year.[4] The percentage reduction varies between and within budget accounts depending on the categories of funding, as described below, contained within each budget account.

After accounting for each category of funding within a budget account, sequestration reductions are spread evenly across all budget account subcomponents referenced in committee reports, budget justifications, and/or Presidential Detailed Budget Estimates – also known as programs, projects or activities. For budget accounts that contain only one category of funding, all sequestrable funds are reduced by the corresponding percentage. For accounts that contain multiple categories of funding, the total amount of each category of sequestrable funds is reduced by its corresponding percentage. The reduced budget resources are usually permanently cancelled.[5]

As currently used, a sequester applies to either discretionary or mandatory spending. Discretionary spending is associated with most funds provided by annual appropriations acts. While all discretionary spending is subject to the annual appropriations process, only a portion of mandatory spending is provided in appropriations acts.[6] Mandatory spending is generally provided by permanent laws, such as the Social Security Act, which made indefinite budget authority permanently available for

---

[4] Sequestration does not apply to every account, since many budget accounts are either exempted from sequestration or governed by special rules under sequestration, the latter of which can vary depending on the sequestration trigger. See BBEDCA §255 and §256, as amended. Since OMB is responsible for the execution and legal interpretations of sequestration orders, some accounts not listed in these sections may also be exempt from sequestration. For a complete list of exempted accounts, see archived CRS Report R42050, *Budget "Sequestration" and Selected Program Exemptions and Special Rules*, coordinated by Karen Spar.

[5] "In some circumstances current law allows for budget authority sequestered in one fiscal year to become available to the agencies again in a subsequent fiscal year. OMB refers to these amounts as 'pop ups.'" See U.S. Government Accountability Office, *2014 Sequestration Opportunities Exist to Improve Transparency of Progress Toward Deficit Reduction Goals*, GAO-16-263, April 2016, p. 27, https://www.gao.gov/assets/680/676565.pdf.

[6] Some mandatory entitlements are provided through the annual appropriations process and are considered "appropriated entitlements" (i.e., Medicaid). Although these entitlements are appropriated, the federal government is legally obligated to make payments to those deemed eligible for the entitlement.

Medicare benefit payments.[7] Some federal programs, such as Medicare, can receive both discretionary and mandatory funding.

In the event that a sequester is triggered, the Office of Management and Budget (OMB) is responsible for calculating the across-the-board percentage reductions, and calculates separate percentages for Medicare, non-defense, and defense funding.[8] Due to sequestration rules, which are covered later in this report, mandatory Medicare benefit payments receive a specific percentage reduction different than other types of federal spending.

The methodologies used to calculate these percentages and the sequestered amounts are published in a report produced by OMB. Once the President issues a sequestration order, the associated report is made available to the public and transmitted to Congress.[9]

Budget Enforcement Rules

Currently, there are three budget enforcement rules that can trigger sequestration. Two were established by the BCA and one was established by Statutory PAYGO. The three rules and their corresponding sequesters can be summarized as follows (and are presented in Table 1):

---

[7] Indefinite budget authority is federal spending that, at the time of enactment, is for an unspecified amount that will be determined at a later date. See U.S. Government Accountability Office, *A Glossary of Terms Used in the Federal Budget Process*, GAO-05-734SP, September 1, 2005, p. 23, https://www.gao.gov/assets/80/76911.pdf.

[8] All funds are first classified as discretionary or mandatory. Within each of these categories, funds are further classified as either Medicare, defense or non-defense. During a sequestration order, each subcomponent of discretionary and/or mandatory funds receives a sequestration percentage based on the necessary amount of savings for that category. For sequestration purposes, Medicare benefit payments are defined by BBEDCA as all payments for programs and activities under Title XVIII of the Social Security Act. See BBEDCA §256(d). Defense and non-defense are referred to in BBEDCA as either "revised security" or "revised nonsecurity," respectively. "Revised security" is any funding coded with a budget function of 050, which is effectively the Department of Defense. "Revised nonsecurity" includes all other government spending. Each of these categories receives a different percentage reduction under a sequestration order.

[9] For more information about the methodologies associated with calculating the sequester percentage in a given year, see *OMB Report to the Congress on the Joint Committee Reductions for Fiscal Year 2018*, May 23, 2017.

Table 1. Medicare Budget Enforcement Rules Summary

Funding Types	Medicare Programs	Sequester	Enforcement Rule	Sequester Percentage Cap	Current Status
Mandatory	Parts A, B, C, and D Benefits; MIP HCFAC; Non-MIP HCFAC; Administration	Statutory PAYGO	If revenue and/or mandatory spending legislation that projects to increase the deficit over a five- and/or 10- year period is enacted, a sequester of certain mandatory spending would be ordered.	4% for benefit payments and MIP HCFAC. None for other spending.	Current law but not triggered.
		BCA Mandatory Sequester	If the Joint Select Committee was unsuccessful at reducing the federal deficit by $1.5 trillion from FY2012-FY2021, mandatory sequestration would be implemented and discretionary limits would be established (with any breaches enforced through sequestration).	2% for benefit payments and MIP HCFAC. None for other spending.[a]	Currently triggered through FY2027.[b]
Discretionary	Non-MIP HCFAC, Administration	BCA Discretionary Sequester		None.	Discretionary limits currently in place through FY2021 but sequester not currently triggered.[c]

Notes: Programs that appear in both categories are funded using mandatory and discretionary funding. In addition to the Medicare sequestration cap, other sequestration rules prohibit sequestration effects from being included in the determination of adjustments to Medicare payment rates, and explicitly exempt Part D low-income subsidies, Part D catastrophic subsidies (reinsurance) and Qualified Individual premiums from sequestration. BCA refers to Budget Control Act. Discretionary Administration includes amounts for payments to contractors to process providers' claims, beneficiary outreach and education, and maintenance of Medicare's information technology infrastructure. HCFAC refers to the Health Care Fraud and Abuse Control Program and is funded through discretionary and mandatory resources and is responsible for activities that fight health care fraud and waste. Mandatory Administration includes amounts for quality improvement organizations and Part B premium payments for Qualifying Individuals. Medicare Benefit Payments are defined by BBEDCA as all payments for programs and activities under Title XVIII of Social Security Act, including the Medicare Integrity Program. MIP HCFAC refers to the Medicare Integrity Program, which focuses on combating fraud in Medicare. Non-MIP HCFAC refers to all HCFAC spending other than MIP.

a The Bipartisan Budget Act of 2018 (BBA 2018; P.L. 115-123) specifies that the non-administrative Medicare sequester percentage cap under the BCA mandatory sequester will be 4% during the first six months of the FY2027 sequestration order and 0% for the next six months of the order. See BBEDCA §251A(6)(C).

b The Bipartisan Budget Act of 2013 (BBA 2013; P.L. 113-67) extended the BCA mandatory sequester through FY2023. A law modifying the COLA for certain military retirees (P.L. 113-82) extended the sequester through FY2024. The Bipartisan Budget Act of 2015 (BBA 2015; P.L. 114-74) extended the sequester through FY2025. BBA 2018 extended the sequester through FY2027.

c BBA 2013 raised the caps under the BCA on defense and non-defense discretionary spending in FY2014 and FY2015. BBA 2015 raised the discretionary spending caps in FY2016 and FY2017. BBA 2018 raised the discretionary caps in FY2018 and FY2019.

Budget Control Act

The BCA established a bipartisan Joint Select Committee on Deficit Reduction (Joint Committee), which was responsible for developing legislation that would reduce the deficit by at least $1.5 trillion from FY2012 to FY2021.[61] However, the Joint Committee was unable to achieve this goal; therefore, Congress and the President were unable to enact corresponding deficit reduction legislation by a date specified in the law. As a result, two types of spending reductions were automatically triggered.[62]

One automatic spending reduction involved the sequestration of certain *mandatory* spending from FY2013 to FY2021. Through subsequent legislation, Congress extended this reduction through FY2027.[63] (This reduction is referred to in this report as the "BCA mandatory sequester").

Additionally, the BCA established statutory limits on *discretionary* spending for FY2013- FY2021.[64] These discretionary spending limits (discretionary caps) restrict the amount of spending permitted through the annual appropriations process for defense and non-defense programs. Any breach of these discretionary caps results in the sequestration of non-exempt discretionary funding. (This reduction is referred to in this report as the "BCA discretionary sequester.") This was triggered once in FY2013

---

[61] See Title IV of the BCA.
[62] See archived CRS Report R42050, *Budget "Sequestration" and Selected Program Exemptions and Special Rules*, coordinated by Karen Spar.
[63] Four subsequent pieces of legislation have extended the BCA mandatory sequester. The Bipartisan Budget Act of 2013 (BBA 2013;) extended the sequester through FY2023. A law modifying the COLA for certain military retirees () extended the sequester through FY2024. The Bipartisan Budget Act of 2015 (BBA 2015;) extended the sequester through FY2025. The Bipartisan Budget Act of 2018 (BBA 2018; H.R. 1892) extended the sequester through FY2027.
[64] Four subsequent pieces of legislation have modified the BCA discretionary caps as enacted. The American Taxpayer Relief Act (ATRA; P.L. 112-240) postponed the start of the FY2013 sequester, until March 1, 2013, and canceled the first two months of spending cuts. BBA 2013 raised the discretionary caps under the BCA on defense and non-defense discretionary spending in FY2014 and FY2015. BBA 2015 raised the discretionary caps in FY2016 and FY2017. BBA 2018 raised the discretionary caps in FY2018 and FY2019. For more information about the discretionary spending limits established under the BCA, see CRS Report R42506, *The Budget Control Act of 2011 as Amended: Budgetary Effects*, by Grant A. Driessen and Marc Labonte.

and can be triggered again if discretionary caps are breached in any fiscal year through FY2021.

Statutory PAYGO

The Statutory PAYGO Act intended to prevent increases in the deficit over a five- and/or 10-year period. If such legislation were to become law, a sequester of certain *mandatory* spending would be ordered. This budget enforcement rule does not have a sunset date and therefore remains in effect under current law. (This reduction is referred to in this report as "Statutory PAYGO sequester").

Although Congress has passed legislation that has been estimated to increase the deficit since the law went into effect, the Statutory PAYGO sequester has never been triggered due to the fact that Congress has voted to prohibit the effects of specific legislation from being counted under Statutory PAYGO. A recent example of this is the Bipartisan Budget Act of 2018 (BBA 2018; P.L. 115-123), which included language to reduce the "scorecards" tallying the total impact of legislation on the deficit to zero.

MEDICARE OVERVIEW

Medicare, which is a federal program that pays for certain health care services of qualified beneficiaries, is subject to sequestration, although special rules limit the extent to which it is impacted. Due to the varying payment structures of the four parts of the program, sequestration is applied differently across Medicare.

Medicare was established in 1965 under Title XVIII of the Social Security Act to provide hospital and supplementary medical insurance to Americans age 65 and older. Over time, the program has been expanded to also include certain disabled persons, including those with end-stage renal disease. In 2017, the program covered an estimated 58 million persons (49 million aged and 9 million disabled).[65]

The Congressional Budget Office (CBO) estimates that total Medicare spending will be about $718 billion in FY2018 and will increase to about $1,390 billion in FY2027.[66] Almost all Medicare spending is mandatory spending that is primarily used to cover benefit payments (i.e., payments to health care providers for their services), administration, and the Medicare Integrity Program (MIP). The remaining Medicare outlays are discretionary and used almost entirely for other administrative activities that are described in more detail later in this report.

Medicare consists of four distinct parts:

1) **Part A** (Hospital Insurance, or HI) covers inpatient hospital services, skilled nursing care, hospice care, and some home health services. Most persons aged 65 and older are automatically entitled to premium-free Part A because they or their spouse paid Medicare payroll taxes for at least 40 quarters (10 years) on earnings covered by either the Social Security or the Railroad Retirement systems. Part A services are paid for out of the Hospital Insurance Trust Fund, which is mainly funded by a dedicated 2.9% payroll tax on earnings of current workers, shared equally between employers and workers.
2) **Part B** (Supplementary Medical Insurance, or SMI) covers a broad range of medical services, including physician services, laboratory services, durable medical equipment, and outpatient hospital services. Enrollment in Part B is optional, but most beneficiaries with Part A also enroll in Part B. Part B benefits are paid for out of the Supplementary Insurance Trust Fund, which is primarily funded through beneficiary premiums and federal general revenues.

---

[65] HHS, *Fiscal Year 2018 Budget in Brief: Putting America's Health First*, 2017, p. 52, at https://www.hhs.gov/sites/ default/files/Consolidated%20BIB_ONLINE_remediated.pdf.

[66] Congressional Budget Office, June 2017 Medicare Baseline, https://www.cbo.gov/sites/default/files/recurringdata/51302-2017-06-medicare.pdf.

3) **Part C** (Medicare Advantage, or MA) is a private plan option that covers all Parts A and B services, except hospice. Individuals choosing to enroll in Part C must be eligible for Part A and must also enroll in Part B. About one-third of Medicare beneficiaries are enrolled in MA. Part C is funded through both the HI and SMI trust funds.
4) **Part D** is a private plan option that covers outpatient prescription drug benefits. This portion of the program is optional. About 76% of Medicare beneficiaries are enrolled in Medicare Part D or have coverage through an employer retiree plan subsidized by Medicare. Part D benefits are paid for out of the Supplementary Insurance Trust Fund, which is primarily funded through beneficiary premiums and federal general revenues.

Beneficiary Costs

Beneficiaries are responsible for paying Medicare Parts B and D premiums, as well as other out-of-pocket costs, such as deductibles and coinsurance,[67] for services provided under all parts of the Medicare program.[68] Under Medicare Parts A, B and D, there is no limit on beneficiary out-of-pocket spending, and most beneficiaries have some form of supplemental insurance through private Medigap plans, employer-sponsored retiree plans, or Medicaid to help cover a portion of their Medicare premiums and/or deductibles and coinsurance. Medicare Advantage has limits on out-of-pocket spending.

---

[67] A deductible is the amount an enrollee is required to pay for health care services or products before his or her insurance plan begins to provide coverage. Coinsurance is the percentage share that an enrollee in a health insurance plan pays for a product or service covered by the plan.
[68] Beneficiaries enrolled in a Medicare Advantage (MA: Part C) plan must pay Part B premiums as well as any additional premium required by the MA plan.

Provider and Plan Payments

Under Medicare Parts A and B, the government generally pays providers directly for services on a *fee-for-service* basis using different prospective payment systems and fee schedules.[69] Under Parts C and D, Medicare pays private insurers a monthly *capitated* per person amount to provide coverage to enrollees, regardless of the amount of services used. The capitated payments are adjusted to reflect differences in the relative cost of sicker beneficiaries with different risk factors including age, disability, or end-stage renal disease.

Health Care Fraud and Abuse Control Program

The Health Care Fraud and Abuse Control Program (HCFAC) was established by the Health Insurance Portability and Accountability Act (HIPAA; P.L. 104-191) and is responsible for activities that fight health care fraud and waste. HCFAC is funded using both mandatory and discretionary funds and consists of three programs: (1) the HCFAC program, which finances the investigative and enforcement activities undertaken by the Department of Health and Human Services (HHS), the HHS Office of Office of Inspector General, the Department of Justice, and the Federal Bureau of Investigation, (2) Medicaid Oversight, and (3) MIP.

Historically, MIP has focused on combating fee-for-service fraud in Medicare Parts A and B. However, increases in private Medicare enrollment—Parts C and D—have expanded program integrity efforts into capitated payment systems as well.

---

[69] Under a *prospective payment system* (PPS), Medicare payments are made using a predetermined, fixed amount based on the classification system for a particular service. The Centers for Medicare and Medicaid Services uses separate PPSs to reimburse acute inpatient hospitals, home health agencies, hospice, hospital outpatient departments, inpatient psychiatric facilities, inpatient rehabilitation facilities, long-term care hospitals, and skilled nursing facilities. A *fee schedule* is a listing of fees used by Medicare to pay doctors or other providers/suppliers. Fee schedules are used to pay for physician services; ambulance services; clinical laboratory services; and durable medical equipment, prosthetics, orthotics, and supplies in certain locations.

While HCFAC is not a part of the Medicare program, MIP is authorized by the same title of the Social Security Act as Medicare and focuses entirely on the program. As a result, this portion of HCFAC is treated as a part of Medicare benefit payments under a sequestration order and would be subject to the Medicare mandatory sequestration percentage limits.[70]

Administrative Spending

The administration of Medicare is funded through a combination of discretionary and mandatory resources that are subject to reductions under a discretionary or mandatory sequestration order, respectively. Discretionary administration funding includes amounts for payments to contractors to process providers' claims, beneficiary outreach and education, and maintenance of Medicare's information technology infrastructure. Mandatory administration funding includes amounts for quality improvement organizations and Part B premium payments for Qualifying Individuals (QI).

MEDICARE SEQUESTRATION RULES

Special rules limit the total effect of budget sequestration on Medicare, as mentioned in Table 1. Most notably, BBEDCA, as amended by the BCA, prohibits Medicare benefit payments from being reduced by more than 2% under a BCA mandatory sequestration order. Similarly, Statutory PAYGO prohibits Medicare benefit payments from being reduced by more than 4% under a Statutory PAYGO sequestration order.[71] The cap does not apply to Medicare mandatory and discretionary administrative spending,

---

[70] For sequestration purposes, BBEDCA defines Medicare benefit payments as all payments for programs and activities under Title XVIII of Social Security Act. This includes MIP. See BBEDCA §256(d).

[71] Medicare benefit payments are considered mandatory budgetary resources and would not be subject to a BCA discretionary sequestration order.

which is subject to the unrestricted percentage reduction under both BCA and Statutory PAYGO sequestration orders.

Under the current mandatory sequestration order triggered by the BCA, the Medicare sequestration percentage is capped at 2%.[72] Therefore, as OMB determines the percentage reductions for each budget category through FY2027, Medicare benefit payments cannot be reduced by more than 2%; as such, another budget category may be subject to a higher percentage reduction in order to achieve the necessary amount of savings.

More specifically, if OMB determines that total non-exempt, non-defense mandatory funds need to be reduced by a percentage larger than 2% in order to achieve necessary savings under a BCA sequestration order for a given year, then a 2% reduction would be made to Medicare benefit spending, and the uniform reduction percentage for the remaining non-Medicare benefit, non-exempt, non-defense mandatory programs would be recalculated and increased by an amount to achieve the necessary level of reductions. If the uniform percentage reduction needed to achieve the total amount of savings is less than 2%, then the determined percentage would be applied to all non-exempt, non-defense, mandatory accounts, including Medicare. Of note, if a mandatory sequestration order were triggered by Statutory PAYGO, the process would be the same, but the reduction of payments for Medicare benefits would be capped at 4%.[73]

In addition to these percentage caps, BBEDCA also prohibits Statutory PAYGO and BCA mandatory sequestration effects from being included in the determination of annual adjustments to Medicare payment rates established under Title XVIII of the Social Security Act.[74] (See "Reductions in Benefit Spending").

Finally, certain Medicare programs and activities are explicitly exempted from Statutory PAYGO and BCA sequestration orders.

---

[72] See BBEDCA §251A(6). In addition, the Bipartisan Budget Act of 2018 (H.R. 1892) specifies that the non-administrative Medicare sequester percentage cap will be 4% during the first 6 months of the FY2027 sequestration order and 0% for the next 6 months of the order. See BBEDCA §251A(6)(C) and Footnote a in Table 1.

[73] See BBEDCA §256(d)(2).

[74] See BBEDCA §256(d)(6).

Specifically, Part D low-income subsidies,[75] Part D catastrophic subsidies (reinsurance),[76] and QI premiums[77] cannot be reduced under a mandatory sequestration order.[78]

MEDICARE SEQUESTER EXECUTION

Timing

Once a sequester is triggered, OMB issues a sequestration order for, at most, one fiscal year, and subsequent orders are reissued for each fiscal year, as necessary. These orders can be issued either before or during the fiscal year in which they apply, depending on the trigger.

Reductions in budget resources are to be made during the effective period of a sequestration order; however special rules differentiate when a sequestration order is implemented for benefit payments. As a result, sequestration orders are applied to Medicare benefit payments on a different timeline than other mandatory and discretionary Medicare funds (i.e., Medicare administration and HCFAC).

Once OMB issues a sequestration order, Medicare benefit payments are sequestered beginning on the first date of the following month and remain in effect for all services furnished during the following one-year period.[79] In the event that a subsequent sequester order is issued prior to the completion of the first order, the subsequent order begins on the first day after the initial order has been completed.

---

[75] Medicare Part D provides subsidies to assist low-income beneficiaries with premiums and cost sharing. For more information on Medicare Part D, see CRS Report R40611, *Medicare Part D Prescription Drug Benefit*, by Suzanne M. Kirchhoff.

[76] Part D plan sponsors pay nearly all drug costs above a catastrophic threshold, except for nominal beneficiary cost sharing. Medicare subsidizes 80% of each plan's costs for this catastrophic coverage. For more information on Medicare Part D, see CRS Report R40611, *Medicare Part D Prescription Drug Benefit*, by Suzanne M. Kirchhoff.

[77] The QI program is a state program that helps pay Part B premiums for people who have Part A and limited income and resources. See Centers for Medicare & Medicaid Services, *Medicare Savings Programs,* https://www.medicare.gov/your-medicare-costs/help-paying-costs/medicare-savings-program/medicare-savingsprograms.html.

[78] See BBEDCA §256(d)(7).

[79] See BBEDCA §256(d)(1).

As an example, the first BCA mandatory sequester order (FY2013) was issued on March 1, 2013, and took effect April 1, 2013. It remained in effect through March 31, 2014. The FY2014 order was issued on April 10, 2013, (corrected on May 20, 2013) and was in effect from April 1, 2014, to March 31, 2015.[80]

All other sequestrable funding is reduced only during the fiscal year associated with the sequester report. Using the same example, the first BCA mandatory sequester order (FY2013) reduced appropriate administrative spending from March 1, 2013, to September 30, 2013. The second order for FY2014 sequestered funds from October 1, 2013, to September 30, 2014.

While OMB uses current law to determine the amount of funds available to be sequestered and corresponding percentage reductions, actual Medicare outlays will not be known until after the end of the fiscal year. Since sequestration orders are issued either before or during the fiscal year in which they are applicable, OMB *estimates* the total sequestrable budget authority for Medicare, and other accounts with indefinite budget authority, in order to determine necessary sequestration percentages.[81]

If Medicare outlays exceed the estimated amount included in a sequestration order for that fiscal year, the additional outlays are sequestered at the established percentage for that fiscal year. If Medicare outlays are determined to be less than the estimated amount, no adjustments are made to the sequestration order. In other words, OMB does not adjust sequestration percentages for any category of budget authority once actuals are realized for accounts with indefinite budget authority. Similarly, OMB does not adjust future orders to account for any previous discrepancies between estimates and actuals.

---

[80] Under current law, the sequestration of Medicare benefits under the BCA is scheduled to continue through September 30, 2027, due to special rules that cap the Medicare sequester percentage at 0% during the last six months of the FY2027 order. Without this rule, Medicare benefit payments would be reduced from April 1, 2027 – March 31, 2028. See BBEDCA §251A(6)(C).

[81] U.S. Government Accountability Office, *2014 Sequestration Opportunities Exist to Improve Transparency of Progress Toward Deficit Reduction Goals*, GAO-16-263, April 2016, p. 27, https://www.gao.gov/assets/680/676565.pdf.

Reductions in Benefit Spending

Parts A and B

Under Medicare Parts A and B, participating providers, such as hospitals and physicians, are paid by the federal government on a fee-for-service basis for services provided to a beneficiary. According to guidance issued by the Centers for Medicare & Medicaid Services (CMS), any sequestration reductions are to be made to claims after determining coinsurance, deductibles, and any applicable Medicare Secondary Payment adjustments.[82] Therefore, sequestration applies only to the portion of the payment paid to providers by Medicare; the beneficiary cost-sharing amounts and amounts paid by other insurance are not reduced.

As an example, if the total allowed payment for a particular service is $100 and the beneficiary has a 20% co-insurance, the beneficiary would be responsible for paying the provider the full $20 in co-insurance. The remaining 80% that is paid by Medicare would be reduced by 2% under the FY2018 sequestration order, or $1.60 in this example, resulting in a total Medicare payment of $78.40. In total, the provider would receive a payment of $98.40. This reduced payment is considered payment in full and the Medicare beneficiary is not expected to pay higher copayments to make up for the reduced Medicare payment.[83]

Part A inpatient services are considered to be furnished on the date of the individual's discharge from the inpatient facility. For services paid on a reasonable cost basis,[84] the reduction is to be applied to payments for such services incurred at any time during each cost reporting period during the sequestration period, for the portion of the cost reporting period that occurs during the effective period of the order. For Part B services provided under

---

[82] Centers for Medicare & Medicaid Services, Medicare FFS Provider e-News, March 8, 2013, *Monthly Payment Reductions in the Medicare Fee-for-Service (FFS) Program – "Sequestration,"* https://www.cms.gov/outreach-andeducation/outreach/ffsprovpartprog/downloads/2013-03-08-standalone.pdf.

[83] Ibid.

[84] Most providers are paid under a prospective payment system or fee schedule. Some types of providers, such as Critical Access Hospitals, are paid on a reasonable cost basis under which payments are based on actual costs incurred. Reasonable cost is defined at Social Security Act §1861(v).

assignment,[85] the reduced payment is to be considered *payment in full* and the Medicare beneficiary will not pay higher copayments to make up for the reduced amount.[86]

Medicare *non-participating* providers, which are providers that do not elect to accept Medicare payments on *all* claims in a given year, are not subject to the same rules. Medicare nonparticipating providers receive a lower reimbursement rate from Medicare on all services provided and may charge beneficiaries a limited amount more (balance bill charge) than the fee schedule amount on non-assigned claims.[87] In these instances, instead of the Medicare check being sent to the provider, a check that incorporates the 2% reduction is mailed to the patient. The patient must then pay the provider an amount that incorporates the sequestered amount. More specifically, as payment, the beneficiary is responsible for paying the provider the amount listed on the check, any cost sharing, balance bill charges, *and* the sequestered amounts taken out of the provider check.[88]

Annual adjustments to Medicare payment rates are determined without incorporating sequestration.[89] However, the Medicare Payment Advisory Commission does incorporate the effects of sequestration when assessing the adequacy of provider payments.[90] The commission uses these annual assessments to develop payment adjustment recommendations to the HHS Secretary and/or Congress.

---

[85] Assignment is an agreement by a doctor, provider, or supplier to be paid directly by Medicare, to accept the payment amount Medicare approves for the service, and not to bill the beneficiary for any more than the Medicare deductible and coinsurance (if applicable). Providers that don't accept assignment may charge more than the Medicare-approved amount.

[86] See CMS, Medicare FFS Provider e-News, March 8, 2013, *Monthly Payment Reductions in the Medicare Fee-forService (FFS) Program – "Sequestration,"* http://www.cms.gov/Outreach-and-Education/Outreach/FFSProvPartProg/Downloads/2013-03-08-standalone.pdf.

[87] Centers for Medicare & Medicaid Services, Frequently Asked Questions, *How does Medicare pay for services delivered by non-participating providers?*, https://questions.cms.gov/faq.php?id=5005&faqId=9920.

[88] CMS, Medicare FFS Provider e-News, March 8, 2013, *Monthly Payment Reductions in the Medicare Fee-for-Service (FFS) Program – "Sequestration,"* https://www.cms.gov/outreach-and-education/outreach/ffsprovpartprog/downloads/ 2013-03-08-standalone.pdf.

[89] BBEDCA Section 256(d)(6).

[90] Medicare Payment Advisory Commission (MedPAC), *Medicare Payment Policy Report to Congress*, March 2017, pp. 57-58, http://medpac.gov/docs/default-source/reports/mar17_entirereport.pdf.

Part C

Under Medicare Advantage, private health plans are paid a per person monthly amount to provide all Medicare-covered benefits, except hospice, to beneficiaries who enroll in their plan. These capitated monthly payments are made to MA plans regardless of how many or how few services beneficiaries actually use. The plan is at risk if costs for all of its enrollees exceed program payments and beneficiary cost sharing; conversely, the plan can generally retain savings if aggregate enrollee costs are less than program payments and cost sharing.

With respect to sequestration, reductions are uniformly made to the monthly capitated payments to the private plans administering Medicare Advantage (Medicare Advantage Organizations or MAOs). These fixed payments are determined every year with CMS approval through an annual "bid process" and the amounts can vary depending on the private plan.[91]

In general, CMS payments to MAOs are generally comprised of amounts to cover medical costs, administrative expenses, private plan profits, risk adjustments, and plan rebates to beneficiaries.[92] MAOs have discretion to distribute any sequestration cut across these four different components but must still adhere to their legal obligations.[93]

Some MAOs have attempted to pass the reduction in their capitation rates onto providers through lower reimbursement rates; however MAOs may be limited in their ability to do so.[94] CMS provided instructions regarding the treatment of contract and non-contract providers that provide

---

[91] For more information on the annual bid process, see CRS Report R44766, *Medicare Advantage (MA)–Proposed Benchmark Update and Other Adjustments for CY2018: In Brief*, by Paulette C. Morgan.

[92] A plan rebate is the difference between a plan's bid and a CMS defined benchmark amount. It is included in the plan payment and must be returned to enrollees in the form of additional benefits, reduced cost sharing, reduced Medicare Part B or Part D premiums, or some combination of these options.

[93] See ay 1, 2013, memorandum from Cheri Rice and Danielle Moon, CMS, *Additional Information Regarding the Mandatory Payment Reductions in the Medicare Advantage, Part D, and Other Programs.* https://www.cms.gov/ Medicare/Medicare-Advantage/Plan-Payment/Downloads/PaymentReductions.pdf.

[94] As a result of the initial BCA sequester, some MAOs attempted to reduce provider payments by 2%. The courts ultimately determined that MAOs were subject to the terms in the contracts with providers. See *Baptist Hosp. of Miami, Inc. v. Humana Health Ins. Co. of Florida, Inc.* and *Butler Healthcare Providers et al. v. Highmark Inc. et al.*

services under Part C. Specifically, "whether and how sequestration might affect an MAO's payments to its contracted providers are governed by the terms of the contract between the MAO and the provider."[95] Therefore, in order for MAOs to reduce provider payments by the sequestered amount, specific language within a contract must allow the reduction or the contract would need to be renegotiated.

In certain instances, such as when beneficiaries receive emergency out-of-network care, MAOs need to reimburse the non-contracted providers; in such cases, the MAOs are required to pay at least the rate providers would have received if the beneficiaries had been enrolled in original Medicare. However, MAOs have the discretion whether or not to incorporate sequestration cuts into payments to non-contracted providers for those services.[96] Non-contracted providers must accept any payments reduced by the sequestration percentage as payment in full.

In addition, regulations in the annual bid process restrict MAO's potential responses to sequestration. Specifically, MAOs are limited to "reasonable" revenue margins and a set Medicare/non-Medicare profit margin discrepancy, among other requirements.[97] Furthermore, MAOs are restricted from allowing sequestration to impact a beneficiary's plan benefits or liabilities,[98] so it becomes difficult for MAOs to pass an entire sequestration cut onto beneficiaries through higher premiums or seek to offset lost revenue by increasing non-Medicare profits.

As HHS computes annual adjustments to Medicare payment rates, the Secretary cannot take into account any reductions in payment amounts under sequestration for the Part C growth percentage.[99] In other words,

---

[95] May 1, 2013, memorandum from Cheri Rice and Danielle Moon, CMS, *Additional Information Regarding the Mandatory Payment Reductions in the Medicare Advantage, Part D, and Other Programs.* https://www.cms.gov/Medicare/Medicare-Advantage/Plan-Payment/Downloads/PaymentReductions.pdf.
[96] Ibid.
[97] See Centers for Medicare & Medicaid Services, *Actuarial Bid Training – 2018*, https://www.cms.gov/Medicare/Health-Plans/MedicareAdvtgSpecRateStats/BidTraining2018.html and 42 CFR Part 422, Subpart X.
[98] See Centers for Medicare & Medicaid Services, *User Group Call 05/07/2015*, May 7, 2015, https://www.cms.gov/Medicare/Health-Plans/MedicareAdvtgSpecRateStats/Downloads/ActuarialBidQuestions2016.pdf.
[99] BBEDCA Section 256(d)(6)(A). The Secretary uses an estimate of the growth in overall spending in Medicare when calculating updated payments to MA plans. See CRS Report

plan payment updates are to be determined as if the reductions under sequestration have not taken place. This results in larger annual adjustments as compared to baselines that incorporate sequestration cuts.

Part D

Under Medicare Part D, each plan receives a base capitated monthly payment, called a direct subsidy, which is adjusted to incorporate three risk sharing mechanisms (low-income subsidies, individual reinsurance, and risk corridor payments). While each plan receives the same direct subsidy amount for each enrollee regardless of how many benefits an enrollee actually uses, plans receive different risk sharing adjustments in their monthly payments. With respect to sequestration, reductions are uniformly made only to the direct subsidy amounts. Part D risk sharing adjustments are exempt from sequestration and are therefore not reduced.[100]

Part D also contains a Retiree Drug Subsidy Program, which pays subsidies to qualified employers and union groups that provide prescription drug insurance to Medicare-eligible, retired workers. Instead of a capitated monthly payment, each sponsor receives a federal subsidy at the end of the year to cover a portion of gross prescription drug costs for each retiree during that year. Under this program, sequestration reductions are applied to the annual subsidy amount.[101]

The HHS Secretary is prohibited from taking into account any reductions in payment amounts under sequestration for purposes of computing the Part D annual growth rate.[102]

R44766, *Medicare Advantage (MA)–Proposed Benchmark Update and Other Adjustments for CY2018: In Brief*, by Paulette C. Morgan.

[100] This is different from Medicare Part C risk sharing adjustments, which are included in the capitated payments and are subject to sequestration.

[101] Centers for Medicare & Medicaid Services, "Mandatory Payment Reduction in CMS' Retiree Drug Subsidy Reconciliation Payments," press release, April 19, 2014, https://www.rds.cms.hhs.gov/sites/default/files/webfiles/documents/mandatorypaymentreduction.pdf.

[102] BBEDCA Section 256(d)(6)(B).

HCFAC

As noted, the HCFAC program is not part of Medicare but does receive mandatory and discretionary funds to ensure the programmatic integrity of the Medicare program. Under a BCA sequestration order of mandatory funds, MIP funds are treated as Medicare budget authority and are subject to the 2% sequester limit. HCFAC mandatory funding that does not exclusively address Medicare is reduced by the non-defense mandatory sequester rate, when applicable.

Administrative Expenses

Under either a mandatory or discretionary sequestration order, administrative spending within non-exempt Medicare and HCFAC programs is reduced by the non-defense rate determined by OMB. See Table 2 for past and current non-defense sequester percentages under the BCA mandatory sequester.

Table 2. Mandatory Percentage Reductions under Budget Control Act Sequestration Orders; FY2013–FY2018

	FY2013	FY2014	FY2015	FY2016	FY2017	FY2018
Medicare						
(Benefit Payments and MIP HCFAC)	2.0%	2.0%	2.0%	2.0%	2.0%	2.0%
Non-defense Mandatory						
(Medicare administrative spending and non-MIP HCFAC)	5.1%	7.2%	7.3%	6.8%	6.9%	6.6%
Defense Mandatory	7.9%	9.8%	9.5%	9.3%	9.1%	8.9%

Source: OMB Reports to Congress on the Joint Committee Sequestration for FY2013 to FY2018.

Notes: Defense Mandatory is any funding coded with a budget function of 050, which is effectively the Department of Defense. Medicare Benefit Payments are defined by BBEDCA as all payments for programs and activities under Title XVIII of Social Security Act. The Health Care Fraud and Abuse Control Program (HCFAC) is responsible for activities that fight health care fraud and waste. Non-defense Mandatory includes all other government spending not defined as Medicare or Defense Mandatory. MIP refers to the Medicare Integrity Program, which is under HCFAC and focuses on combating fraud in Medicare.

MEDICARE AND THE BCA MANDATORY SEQUESTER

Since the first BCA mandatory sequester order issued in FY2013, Medicare benefit payments have been subject to the 2% annual reduction limit established by the BCA. Non-defense mandatory budget authority reductions, which have applied to Medicare administrative spending, have fluctuated between 5.1% and 7.3% through FY2018.

In the same sequestration order, Medicare administrative expenses will be sequestered by the non-defense mandatory percentage, 6.6%. The total reduction in Medicare administration budget authority, however, cannot be identified from the data presented in the OMB sequestration report.[103]

In total, Medicare benefit payments (not including administration) are estimated to account for 89% of all Medicare and non-Medicare resources *available* to be sequestered (sequestrable budget authority) under the FY2018 BCA mandatory sequester.[104] Of the funds that are sequestered, Medicare benefit payments are estimated to account for 70% of sequestered funds.[105]

Traditionally, Medicare benefit payments comprise the largest single source of sequestered funds in a given mandatory sequestration order. In FY2018, Medicare benefit payments are estimated to account for the largest share of sequestrable budget authority and sequestered funds since the first BCA sequestration order was issued for FY2013, as shown in Figure 1.[106]

---

[103] CMS receives administrative funding for the Medicare program through the Medicare trust funds and the CMS program management account. Since the *OMB Report to the Congress on the Joint Committee Reductions for Fiscal Year 2018* shows the amount of administrative funding sequestered at the account level, and CMS funds other programs through the program management account, the total amount of administrative funding for the Medicare program cannot be determined from the source.

[104] For a list of sequestrable budget authority by budget account, see *OMB Report to the Congress on the Joint Committee Reductions for Fiscal Year 2018.* May 23, 2017.

[105] Ibid.

[106] Since the mandatory BCA sequester went into effect, the total amount of Medicare benefit payments in a fiscal year has generally increased at a fast rate than other mandatory spending in the corresponding fiscal year. If current trends continue, Medicare benefit payments can be expected to continue to account for larger shares of total sequestered funds through the end of the BCA mandatory sequester in FY2027. In **Figure 1**, Medicare benefit payments constituted a higher percentage of all sequestered funds in FY2013 because the

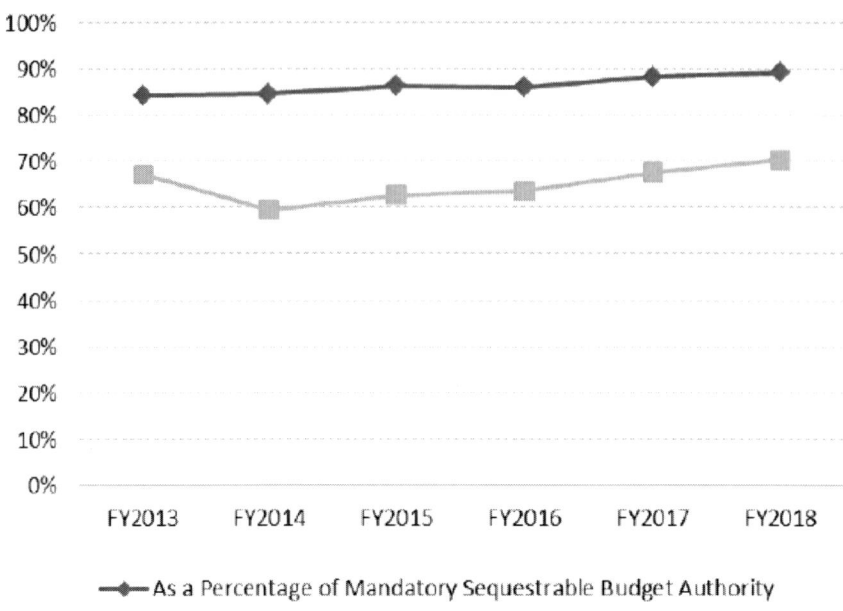

- As a Percentage of Mandatory Sequestrable Budget Authority
- As a Percentage of Mandatory Sequestered Funds

Source: CRS analysis of OMB Reports to the Congress on the Joint Committee Sequestration for FY2013 to FY2018.

Notes: Sequestrable budget authority refers to all resources estimated to be available to be sequestered. Sequestered Funds refers to all resources estimated to be sequestered. Administrative funding is not included in Medicare benefit payment totals. All percentages are estimates.

Figure 1. Medicare Benefit Payments As a Percentage of Budget Control Act Mandatory Sequester Amounts; FY2013-FY2018.

Figure 2 shows how the FY2018 BCA sequestration order is estimated to apply to the various parts of Medicare. It is worth noting that although Medicare Part C is sequestered, OMB sequestration orders delineate at the trust fund level and do not distinguish each Medicare part. Part C is funded

---

American Taxpayer Relief Act of 2012 (P.L. 112 240) reduced the total amount of sequestered funds in FY2013 relative to all other fiscal years under the BCA mandatory sequester.

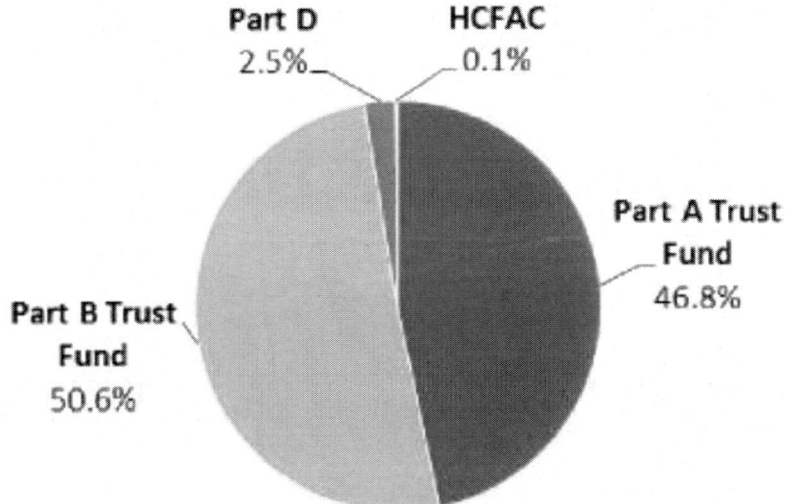

Source: CRS analysis of OMB Report to the Congress on the Joint Committee Reductions for Fiscal Year 2018, May 23, 2017.

Notes: Administrative funding is not included. Although Medicare Part C is sequestered, OMB sequestration orders delineate at the trust fund level and do not distinguish each Medicare part. Part C is funded out of both the Part A and Part B trust funds and is included in these totals.

Figure 2. Estimated Source of Sequestered Medicare Benefits in FY2018; Total Reduction in Medicare Benefit Payments - $12.76 billion.

out of both the Part A and Part B trust funds and is included in these totals. For reference, from FY2016-FY2017, Medicare Advantage, on average, accounted for 32% of all HI Trust Fund benefit payments and 38% of all SMI Trust Fund benefit payments.[107] These ratios could change in FY2018 based on actual spending.

CBO estimates that Medicare benefit payment outlays will increase 96% from FY2018 to FY2027 ($708 billion to $1,387 billion), which is the last year of BCA mandatory sequestration.[108] Most of this expected

---

[107] Centers for Medicare & Medicaid Services, *CMS Financial Report*, FY2017, November 3, 2017, pp. 43-44, https://www.cms.gov/Research-Statistics-Data-and-Systems/Statistics-Trends-and-Reports/CFOReport/Downloads/ 2017_CMS_Financial_Report.pdf.

[108] Congressional Budget Office, June 2017 Medicare Baseline, https://www.cbo.gov/sites/default/files/recurringdata/ 51302-2017-06-medicare.pdf.

increase is due to an aging population and rising health care costs per person. In addition, most of this increase would be subject to sequestration.[109]

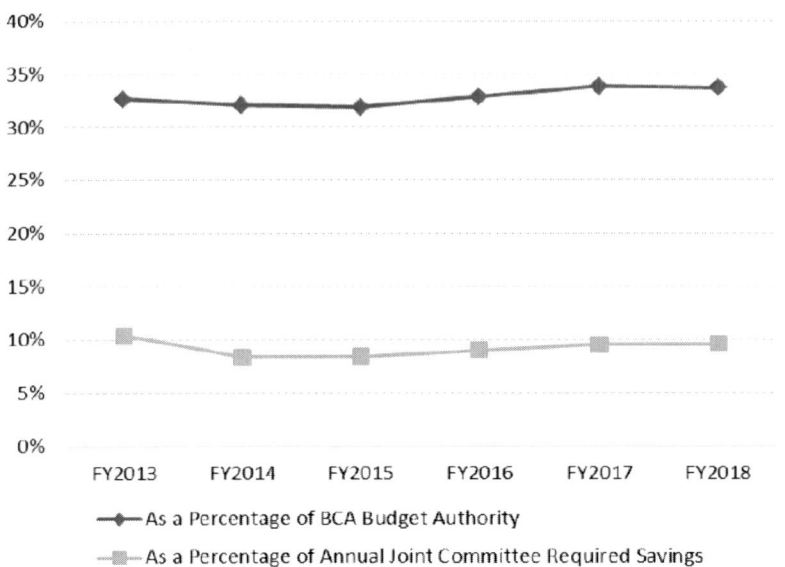

Source: CRS analysis of OMB Reports to the Congress on the Joint Committee Sequestration for FY2013 to FY2018.

Notes: BCA refers to Budget Control Act. BCA Budget Authority refers to all resources used in the baseline to determine discretionary cap savings, mandatory sequestration percentages, and interest. Annual Joint Committee Required Savings refers to all resources reduced by the discretionary caps, sequestered, and interest saved, as determined by OMB. Administrative funding is not included in Medicare benefit payment totals. These percentages are developed from OMB Reports to the Congress on the Joint Committee Sequestration for FY2013 to FY2018. The methodologies included in these reports do not incorporate any increases in discretionary caps associated with BBA 2013, BBA 2015, and BBA 2018. All percentages are estimates.

Figure 3. Medicare Benefit Payment Reductions as a Percentage of Budget Control Act Amounts; Y2013-FY2018.

---

[109] Congressional Budget Office, *The 2017 Long-Term Budget Outlook*, March 2017, https://www.cbo.gov/system/files/ 115th-congress-2017-2018/reports/52480-ltbo.pdf.

When Congress failed to enact legislation that reduced the deficit by at least $1.5 trillion before January 15, 2012, the BCA prompted savings from three sources: (1) the mandatory sequestration of funds, (2) reduced discretionary spending limits, and (3) lower expected interest payments on U.S. government debt, which resulted from the mandatory sequestration of funds and discretionary spending limits. Although Medicare benefit payments traditionally account for a large percentage of mandatory sequestered funds, they account for a much smaller portion of overall BCA savings—generally around 10%—because reduced discretionary spending limits account for a larger share of BCA savings than the mandatory sequester. In FY2018, sequestered Medicare benefit payments will account for approximately 10% of total FY2018 BCA savings, as determined by OMB and shown in Figure 3.[110]

APPENDIX A. BUDGET TERMINOLOGY DEFINITIONS

As defined by Balanced Budget and Emergency Deficit Control Act of 1985 (BBEDCA; P.L. 99 177) and simplified where appropriate:

Budget Authority—Authority provided by federal law to enter into financial obligations that will result in immediate or future outlays involving federal government funds.

Budgetary Resources—An amount available to enter into new obligations and to liquidate them. Budgetary resources are made up of new budget authority (including direct spending authority provided in existing statute and obligation limitations) and unobligated balances of budget authority provided in previous years.

---

[110] These percentages are developed from OMB Reports to the Congress on the Joint Committee Sequestration for FY2013 to FY2018. The methodologies included in these reports do not incorporate any increases in discretionary caps associated with BBA 2013, BBA 2015, and BBA 2018.

Discretionary Appropriations—Budgetary resources (except to fund direct-spending programs) provided in appropriation Acts.

Mandatory Spending—Also known as "direct spending," refers to budget authority that is provided in laws other than appropriation acts, entitlement authority, and the Supplemental Nutrition Assistance Program.

Medicare Benefit Payments—All payments for programs and activities under Title XVIII of the Social Security Act.

Revised Nonsecurity Category—Discretionary appropriations other than in budget function 050.

Revised Security Category—Discretionary appropriations in budget function 050.

Sequestration—The cancellation of budgetary resources provided by discretionary appropriations or direct spending laws.

For definitions of other budget terms mentioned in this report but not defined by BBEDCA, see U.S. Government Accountability Office, *A Glossary of Terms Used in the Federal Budget Process*, GAO-05-734SP, September 1, 2005, p. 23, https://www.gao.gov/assets/80/76911.pdf.

In: Medicare: Financing, Insolvency and Fraud ISBN: 978-1-53614-811-4
Editor: Bradford Rodgers © 2019 Nova Science Publishers, Inc.

Chapter 4

MEDICARE: CMS SHOULD TAKE ACTIONS TO CONTINUE PRIOR AUTHORIZATION EFFORTS TO REDUCE SPENDING[*]

United States Government Accountability Office

WHY GAO DID THIS STUDY

CMS required prior authorization as a demonstration in 2012 for certain power mobility devices, such as power wheelchairs, in seven states. Under the prior authorization process, MACs review prior authorization requests and make determinations to approve or deny them based on Medicare coverage and payment rules. Approved requests will be paid as long as all other Medicare payment requirements are met.

---

[*] This is an edited, reformatted and augmented version of United States Government Accountability Office; Report to the Committee on Finance, U.S. Senate; Accessible Version, Publication No. GAO-18-341, dated April 2018.

United States Government Accountability Office

GAO was asked to examine CMS's prior authorization programs. GAO examined 1) the changes in expenditures and the potential savings for items and services subject to prior authorization demonstrations, 2) reported benefits and challenges of prior authorization, and 3) CMS's monitoring of the programs and plans for future prior authorization. To do this, GAO examined prior authorization program data, CMS documentation, and federal internal control standards. GAO also interviewed CMS and MAC officials, as well as selected provider, supplier, and beneficiary groups.

WHAT GAO RECOMMENDS

GAO recommends that CMS (1) subject accessories essential to the power wheelchairs in the permanent DMEPOS program to prior authorization and (2) take steps, based on results from evaluations, to continue prior authorization. The Department of Health and Human Services neither agreed nor disagreed with GAO's recommendations but said it would continue to evaluate prior authorization programs and take GAO's findings and recommendations into consideration in developing plans or determining appropriate next steps.

WHAT GAO FOUND

Prior authorization is a payment approach used by private insurers that generally requires health care providers and suppliers to first demonstrate compliance with coverage and payment rules before certain items or services are provided to patients, rather than after the items or services have been provided. This approach may be used to reduce expenditures, unnecessary utilization, and improper payments. The Centers for Medicare & Medicaid Services (CMS) has begun using prior authorization in Medicare through a series of fixed-length demonstrations designed to measure their effectiveness, and one permanent program. According to GAO's analyses, expenditures decreased for items and services subject to a demonstration. GAO's analyses of actual expenditures and estimated expenditures in the absence of the demonstrations found that estimated savings from all demonstrations through March 2017 could be as high as about $1.1 to $1.9 billion. While CMS officials said that prior authorization likely played a large role in reducing expenditures, it is difficult to separate the effects of prior authorization from other program integrity efforts. For example, CMS implemented a durable medical equipment competitive bidding program in January 2011, and according to the agency, it resulted in lower expenditures.

Many provider, supplier, and beneficiary group officials GAO spoke with reported benefits of prior authorization, such as reducing unnecessary utilization. However, provider and supplier group officials reported that providers and suppliers experienced some challenges. These include difficulty obtaining the necessary documentation from referring physicians to submit a prior authorization request, although CMS has created templates and other tools to address this concern. In addition, providers and suppliers reported concerns about whether accessories deemed essential to the power wheelchairs under the permanent durable medical equipment, prosthetics, orthotics, and supplies (DMEPOS) program are subject to prior authorization. In practice, Medicare Administrative Contractors (MAC) that administer prior authorization programs review these accessories when making prior authorization determinations, even though they are not technically included in the program and therefore cannot be provisionally affirmed. As a result, providers and suppliers lack assurance about whether Medicare is likely to pay for these accessories. This is contrary to a CMS stated benefit of prior authorization—to provide assurance about whether Medicare is likely to pay for an item or service—and to federal internal control standards, which call for agencies to design control activities that enable an agency to achieve its objectives.

CMS monitors prior authorization through various MAC reports. CMS also reviews MAC accuracy and timeliness in processing prior authorization requests and has contracted for independent evaluations of the demonstrations. Currently, prior authorization demonstrations are scheduled to end in 2018. Despite its interest in using prior authorization for additional items, CMS has not made plans to continue its efforts. Federal internal control standards state that agencies should identify, analyze, and respond to risks related to achieving objectives. CMS risks missed opportunities for achieving its stated goals of reducing costs and realizing program savings by reducing unnecessary utilization and improper payments.

ABBREVIATIONS

CMS	Centers for Medicare & Medicaid Services
DMEPOS	durable medical equipment, prosthetics, orthotics, and supplies
HHS	Department of Health and Human Services
MAC	Medicare Administrative Contractor

441 G St. N.W. Washington,
DC 20548

April 20, 2018
The Honorable Orrin Hatch
Chairman
Committee on Finance United States Senate

Dear Mr. Chairman:

Prior authorization is a payment approach used by private insurers that generally requires health care providers and suppliers to first demonstrate compliance with coverage and payment rules before certain items or services are provided to patients, rather than after the items or services have been provided. This approach may be used to reduce expenditures, unnecessary utilization, and improper payments.[111] The Centers for Medicare & Medicaid Services (CMS)—the agency within the Department of Health and Human Services (HHS) that administers the Medicare program—has begun using prior authorization to help ensure program integrity for selected items and services with high levels of unnecessary utilization and improper payments. In fiscal year 2017, the federal government made an estimated $36.2 billion in improper payments for the Medicare fee-for-service program.[112] Since 1990, we have designated Medicare a high-risk program because of its size, complexity, and susceptibility to mismanagement and improper payments.[113]

CMS required prior authorization as a demonstration in 2012 for certain power mobility devices in seven states. CMS conducts demonstrations to test or measure the effect of program changes, such as new or innovative payment approaches. Since that time, CMS has expanded this demonstration to additional states and implemented three additional demonstrations for other items or services, such as non-emergency hyperbaric oxygen therapy, and established a permanent program for certain types of power wheelchairs.[114] For the purposes of our report, we refer to the demonstrations and the permanent program collectively as prior authorization programs unless otherwise noted.

---

[111] In general, improper payments include payments made in error, such as payments that should not have been made; payments made in incorrect amounts, including overpayments and underpayments; and payments for claims that were not properly documented.

[112] Improper payment estimates are calculated from claims processed from July 2015 to June 2016. Department of Health and Human Services, FY2017 Agency Financial Report (Washington, D.C.: Nov. 14, 2017). Medicare is the federally financed health insurance program for persons aged 65 and over, certain individuals with disabilities, and individuals with end-stage renal disease. Medicare fee-for-service, or original Medicare, consists of Medicare Parts A and B. Medicare Part A covers hospital and other inpatient stays. Medicare Part B is optional insurance and covers physician, outpatient hospital, home health care, certain other services, and the rental or purchase of durable medical equipment, prosthetics, orthotics, and supplies (DMEPOS).

[113] See GAO, *High-Risk Series: Progress on Many High-Risk Areas, While Substantial Efforts Needed on Others*, GAO-17-317 (Washington, D.C.: February 2017).

[114] Hyperbaric oxygen therapy is a treatment in which the entire body is exposed to oxygen under increased atmospheric pressure.

You asked us to review CMS's use of prior authorization in Medicare, including findings from current programs, benefits and challenges, and any opportunities for expansion. This report examines

1) the changes in expenditures and the potential savings for items and services subject to prior authorization demonstrations.
2) the reported benefits and challenges of prior authorization.
3) CMS's monitoring of prior authorization programs and its plans for future prior authorization.

To determine changes in expenditures and the potential savings for items and services subject to prior authorization demonstrations, we analyzed Medicare monthly expenditure data. We did not analyze expenditure data for the permanent program because it was implemented in March 2017. We calculated monthly expenditures for each demonstration for 2 time periods: 1) the 6 months prior to implementation of each demonstration and 2) the start of implementation of each demonstration through March 2017, the month for which the most recent reliable data were available at the time of our analysis. We analyzed these data separately for three groups of states: initial demonstration states (states that were part of the initial implementation), expansion demonstration states (states added after the initial implementation of the demonstration), and non-demonstration states (states that were never part of the demonstration).[115] We calculated average monthly expenditures by state for each of the three groups of states. We then estimated potential savings by comparing average monthly expenditures before and after implementation

---

[115] For each demonstration, we considered the implementation month to be the same for all initial demonstration states. For the power mobility device and repetitive scheduled non-emergency ambulance services demonstrations, CMS increased the number of states covered under the demonstration after the initial implementation. We considered the implementation month to be the same for all expansion demonstration states for each demonstration. Implementation was delayed for the non-emergency hyperbaric oxygen demonstration from March 2015 to July 2015 for two states. CMS refers to the various prior authorization programs as the certain power mobility devices and home health services demonstrations and the repetitive scheduled non-emergent ambulance transport services and non-emergent hyperbaric oxygen models. For the purposes of this report, we refer to all of these as demonstrations.

in initial and expansion demonstration states. For the power mobility device demonstration, we also estimated potential savings from reduced expenditures in non-demonstration states, since CMS officials stated that savings may occur in all states—even those not part of the demonstration—in part because they think that larger nationwide suppliers could have improved their compliance with CMS policies in all states based on their experiences with prior authorization. Finally, we analyzed the effect of prior authorization over time by determining the percentage of the total reduction in expenditures that took place in the first 6 months of implementation for each demonstration.[116] We did not independently verify the accuracy of these data on CMS's Medicare expenditures; however, we checked these data for obvious errors and omissions, compared analyses results to CMS's publicly reported information about expenditures, and interviewed CMS officials to resolve any identified discrepancies. On the basis of these actions, we determined that these data were sufficiently reliable for the purpose of our reporting objectives. We also interviewed CMS officials and reviewed CMS documents, such as CMS's annual program integrity report, to identify other program integrity efforts that may have affected expenditures.

To identify reported benefits and challenges of prior authorization, we interviewed multiple stakeholders. First, we interviewed a non-generalizable sample of officials from nine Medicare beneficiary and provider and supplier groups to learn about their experiences with Medicare prior authorization, including challenges they faced and their views on program benefits. Second, we interviewed officials from CMS and the six Medicare Administrative Contractors (MAC) that administer the Medicare prior authorization programs about program benefits and challenges implementing and conducting the programs. When possible, we reviewed relevant documentation, such as the prior authorization

---

[116] We calculated total expenditures in the 6th month after implementation and total expenditures in March 2017 for initial demonstration states for the repetitive scheduled non-emergency ambulance services, power mobility devices, and non-emergency hyperbaric oxygen therapy demonstrations. We then used these data, as well as average monthly expenditures for the 6 months prior to each demonstration's initial implementation, to determine—from implementation through March 2017—the percentage of the total reduction in expenditures that took place within the first 6 months.

programs' operational guides, to corroborate information reported by stakeholders. Third, we interviewed a sample of four private health insurers and two associations that represent health insurers about their experiences with prior authorization. To identify private health insurers, we considered which insurers had the greatest market share among large group insurers in states with Medicare prior authorization programs and which offered Medicare Advantage plans, as well as whether the insurer had been discussed in stakeholder interviews as having particularly relevant experience.[117] We then compared CMS's efforts to mitigate reported challenges to federal standards for internal controls related to control activities.[118]

To determine the monitoring CMS conducts of prior authorization and its plans for future prior authorization, we obtained and reviewed CMS and Medicare contractor documents including Federal Register notices, proposed and final rules, and CMS prior authorization demonstration status updates. We interviewed CMS officials regarding the agency's monitoring of prior authorization and the extent to which the agency has plans for future prior authorization. We also interviewed private health insurers about their prior authorization programs and the evaluations they conduct, including how they determine whether to add or remove items and services from prior authorization. We then compared CMS's efforts in these areas to identified federal standards for internal control related to risk assessment.[119]

We conducted this performance audit from November 2016 through April 2018 in accordance with generally accepted government auditing standards. Those standards require that we plan and perform the audit to obtain sufficient, appropriate evidence to provide a reasonable basis for our findings and conclusions based on our audit objectives. We believe that the

---

[117] The Medicare Advantage program—also known as Medicare Part C—is the private plan alternative to the traditional Medicare program.

[118] See GAO, *Standards for Internal Control in the Federal Government*, GAO-14-704G (Washington, D.C.: September 2014). Internal control is a process effected by an entity's oversight body, management, and other personnel that provides reasonable assurance that the objectives of an entity will be achieved.

[119] See GAO-14-704G.

evidence obtained provides a reasonable basis for our findings and conclusions based on our audit objectives.

BACKGROUND

Since September 2012, CMS has subjected selected items and services to prior authorization and pre-claim reviews—a process similar to prior authorization where review takes place after services have begun—through four fixed-length demonstrations and a permanent program.[120] The prior authorization demonstrations are for certain power mobility devices, repetitive scheduled non-emergency ambulance services, non-emergency hyperbaric oxygen therapy, and home health services; while the permanent program is for certain durable medical equipment, prosthetics, orthotics, and supplies (DMEPOS) items. By using prior authorization, CMS generally seeks to reduce expenditures, unnecessary utilization, and improper payments, although specific objectives for the programs vary based on the statutory authority CMS used to initiate each.

Medicare Prior Authorization Programs

Power Mobility Devices Demonstration

In September 2012, CMS implemented prior authorization for certain scooters and power wheelchairs, items the agency has identified with historically high levels of fraud and improper payments, for Medicare beneficiaries in seven states: California, Florida, Illinois, Michigan, New York, North Carolina, and Texas. The demonstration, established under Section 402(a) of the Social Security Amendments of 1967, is intended to develop or demonstrate improved methods for the investigation and

---

[120] For the purposes of this report, we refer to prior authorization and pre-claim review as prior authorization.

prosecution of fraud in providing care or services under Medicare.[121] In October 2014, CMS expanded the demonstration to 12 additional states: Arizona, Georgia, Indiana, Kentucky, Louisiana, Maryland, Missouri, New Jersey, Ohio, Pennsylvania, Tennessee, and Washington. CMS also extended the program, which was originally scheduled to end in 2015, until August 2018.

Repetitive Scheduled Non-Emergency Ambulance Services Demonstration

In December 2014, CMS implemented prior authorization for repetitive scheduled non-emergency ambulance services in three states the agency has identified with high utilization and improper payment rates, based on the garage location of the ambulance: New Jersey, Pennsylvania, and South Carolina. A repetitive ambulance service—which is defined as medically necessary ambulance transportation that is furnished three or more times during a 10-day period or at least once per week for at least 3 weeks—is most typically associated with transportation to services like dialysis or chemotherapy, according to CMS officials. According to CMS, previous analysis shows that non-emergency ambulance services to and from dialysis facilities have grown noticeably in recent years and now represent a large share of non-emergency ambulance claims. The demonstration, established under Section 1115A of the Social Security Act, is intended to reduce expenditures while preserving or enhancing quality of care.[122] In January 2016, CMS increased the number of states included in the demonstration in accordance with Section 515(a) of the Medicare Access and CHIP Reauthorization Act of 2015: Delaware, District of Columbia, Maryland, North Carolina, Virginia, and West

---

[121] Pub. L. No. 90-248, § 402(a), 81 Stat. 821, 930 (1968) (codified, as amended, at 42 U.S.C. § 1395b-1(a)(1)(J)).

CMS officials reported that since the prior authorization programs' implementation, the agency made more than 100 referrals to its contractors that investigate fraud. However, due to the length of time fraud investigations typically take, results from these referrals are not yet available.

[122] 42 U.S.C. § 1315a.

Virginia.[123] In December 2017, CMS extended the program, which was originally scheduled to end in 2017, through November 2018.[124]

Non-Emergency Hyperbaric Oxygen Therapy Demonstration

In March 2015, CMS implemented prior authorization for non-emergency hyperbaric oxygen therapy in three states the agency has identified with high utilization and improper payment rates, based on the therapy facility's location: Illinois, Michigan, and New Jersey. Medicare covers hyperbaric oxygen therapy for certain conditions, such as diabetic wounds of the lower extremities, after there have been 30 days of no measurable signs of healing during standard wound care treatment. According to CMS, previous experience indicates that hyperbaric oxygen therapy has a high potential for improper payments and raises concerns about beneficiaries receiving medically unnecessary care. The demonstration, established under Section 1115A of the Social Security Act, is intended to reduce expenditures while preserving or enhancing quality of care. The demonstration ended in February 2018.

Home Health Services Demonstration

In August 2016, CMS implemented prior authorization for home health services in Illinois. The demonstration, established under Section 402(a) of the Social Security Amendments of 1967, is intended to develop or demonstrate improved methods for the investigation and prosecution of fraud in providing care or services under Medicare. The demonstration was originally scheduled to incorporate other states the agency has identified with high rates of fraud and abuse: Florida, Massachusetts, Michigan, and Texas. However, as of April 2017, CMS paused the demonstration while it

---

[123] Pub, L. No. 114-10, § 515(a) 129 Stat. 87, 174 (2015). For purposes of this report, we refer to the increase in the number of states included in the demonstration as a demonstration expansion.

[124] Section 515(b) of the Medicare Access and CHIP Reauthorization Act of 2015 provides that the Secretary shall expand the demonstration nationally if the Secretary determines that such an expansion (1) is expected to reduce spending without reducing quality of care or improve the quality of care without increasing spending, (2) would reduce net program spending, and (3) would not deny or limit Medicare coverage. 42 U.S.C. §§ 1395m(l)(16), 1315a(c).

considered making improvements. As of February 2018, the demonstration has not resumed.

Permanent DMEPOS Program

In December 2015, CMS established a permanent prior authorization program for certain DMEPOS items under Section 1834(a)(15) of the Social Security Act.[125] This program aims to reduce unnecessary utilization for certain DMEPOS items. To select the items that would be subject to prior authorization, CMS compiled a Master List of items that 1) appear on the DMEPOS Fee Schedule list, 2) have an average purchase fee of $1,000 or greater (adjusted annually for inflation) or an average rental fee schedule of $100 or greater (adjusted annually for inflation), and 3) meet one of these two criteria: the item was identified in a GAO or HHS Office of Inspector General report that is national in scope and published in 2007 or later as having a high rate of fraud or unnecessary utilization, or the item is listed in the 2011 or later published Comprehensive Error Rate Testing program's annual report.[126] CMS may choose specific items from this Master List to include on the required prior authorization list, and there is no set end date for requiring prior authorization for those items. CMS may suspend prior authorization for those items at any time. (See app. I for the items on the Master List.) In March 2017, CMS began requiring prior authorization for two types of group 3 power wheelchairs from the Master List for beneficiaries with a permanent address in selected states (Illinois, Missouri, New York, and West Virginia) and expanded the program nationwide in July 2017.[127] As of February 2018, CMS has not identified

---

[125] Section 1834(a)(15) of the Social Security Act authorizes the Secretary to develop and periodically update a list of DMEPOS items that are frequently subject to unnecessary utilization and to develop a prior authorization process for these items. 42 U.S.C. § 1395m(a)(15).

[126] See Medicare Program; Implementation Of Prior Authorization Process for Certain Durable Medical Equipment, Prosthetics, Orthotics, and Supplies (DMEPOS) Items and Publication of the Initial Required Prior Authorization List of DMEPOS Items That Require Prior Authorization as a Condition of Payment, 81 Fed. Reg. 93636 (Dec. 21, 2016). CMS updates the Master List annually. As of February 2018, it included 135 items that have high rates of fraud, unnecessary utilization, or improper payments.

[127] CMS defines group 3 wheelchairs as those that can accommodate complex rehabilitative technology accessories. Group 3 power wheelchairs accommodate beneficiaries with limited mobility due to certain neurological conditions, among other things. The

any other items from the Master List for prior authorization. See Figure 1 for each prior authorization program's implementation and end dates.

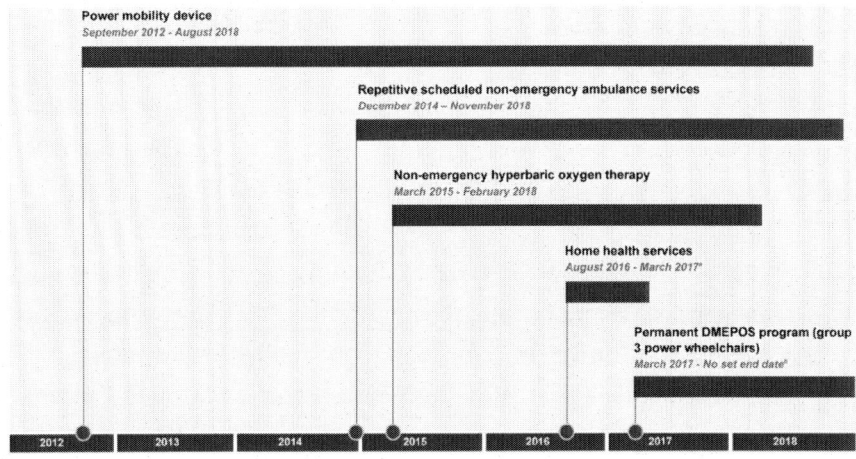

Source: GAO analysis of Centers for Medicare & Medicaid Services information. | GAO-18-341.

ᵃThe home health services demonstration was scheduled to run through July 2019, but the Centers for Medicare & Medicaid Services (CMS) paused the demonstration in April 2017. As of February 2018, the demonstration had not resumed.

ᵇThere is no set end date for requiring prior authorization for these durable medical equipment, prosthetics, orthotics, and supplies (DMEPOS) items. CMS may suspend prior authorization for these items at any time.

Figure 1. Prior Authorization Programs' Implementation and End Dates.

Medicare Prior Authorization Process

MACs that administer the prior authorization programs review prior authorization requests for items and services, along with supporting documentation, to determine whether all applicable Medicare coverage and payment rules have been met. CMS expects requests for prior authorization to include all documentation necessary to show that coverage requirements have been met, for example face-to-face examination documentation or the

---

wheelchairs selected for the permanent DMEPOS program were not included in the power mobility device demonstration.

detailed product description.[128] The referring physician—or the physician who conducts the face-to-face examination of the beneficiary and orders the item or service—provides this documentation to a provider or supplier who subsequently furnishes the item or service. According to multiple MACs' officials, the provider or supplier who furnishes the item or service typically submits the prior authorization request.[129] CMS has specified that MACs review initial prior authorization requests and make a determination within 10 business days.[130] MACs make one of the following decisions:

- Provisionally affirm (approve) – Documentation submitted meets Medicare's coverage and payment rules. A prior authorization provisional affirmation is a preliminary finding that a future claim submitted to Medicare for the item or service meets Medicare's coverage and payment requirements and will likely be paid.[131]
- Non-affirm (deny) – Documentation submitted does not meet Medicare rules or the item or service is not medically necessary. However, a non-affirmed request may be revised and resubmitted for review an unlimited number of times prior to the submission of the claim for payment. CMS has specified that MACs make a determination on a resubmission within 20 business days.

For the demonstrations, claims that are submitted without a prior authorization provisional affirmation are subject to prepayment review, which is medical review before the claim is paid.[132] In addition, for the home health services and power mobility devices demonstrations, claims

---

[128] CMS's documentation requirements did not change under the prior authorization programs.
[129] Beneficiaries may also submit prior authorization requests for the repetitive scheduled non-emergency ambulance service, non-emergency hyperbaric oxygen therapy, and home health services demonstrations; and referring physicians may submit them for the power mobility device demonstration. However, CMS and some of the MACs told us that beneficiaries and referring physicians rarely submit prior authorization requests.
[130] An expedited review process of 2 business days is available for cases where the beneficiary's health could be jeopardized without timely access to the item or service.
[131] Other requirements necessary for payment can only be determined after a claim is submitted, such as proof of delivery of an item or whether it is a duplicate claim.
[132] Medicare claims are typically not subject to medical review, which includes a review of medical records. Less than 1 percent of claims are selected for a medical review.

submitted without a prior authorization provisional affirmation that are determined payable during the medical review will be subject to a 25 percent reduction in payment. For the permanent program, claims that are submitted without a prior authorization provisional affirmation are denied. (See Figure 2 for the prior authorization process.)

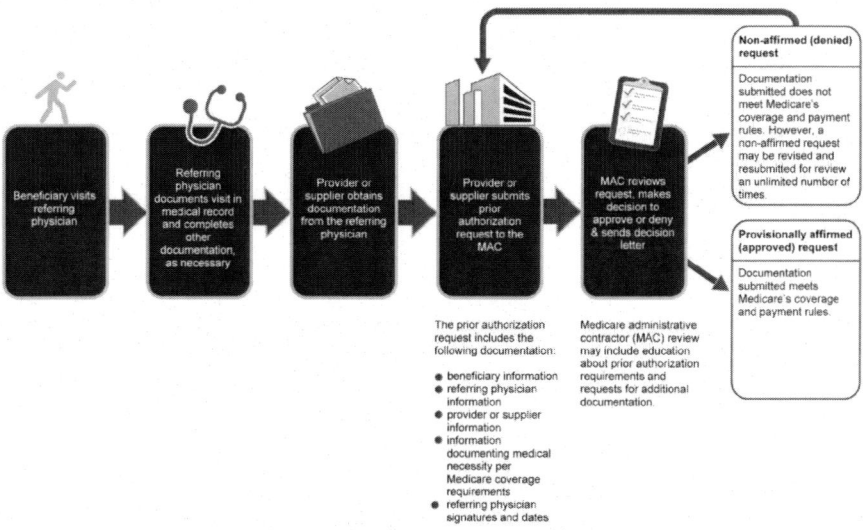

Source: GAO analysis of Centers for Medicare & Medicaid Services information. | GAO-18-341.

Figure 2. Prior Authorization Process.

As of March 31, 2017, MACs had processed over 337,000 prior authorization requests—about 264,000 initial requests and about 73,000 resubmissions, as shown in Table 1.[133]

MACs' provisional affirmation rates for both initial and resubmitted prior authorization requests rose in each demonstration between their implementation and March 2017, often by 10 percentage points or more. For example, the provisional affirmation rate for initial submissions for repetitive scheduled non-emergency ambulance services rose from 28

---

[133] Numbers of decisions do not include 34,976 rejected submissions for all demonstrations. Numbers of decisions for power mobility device demonstration do not include decisions made by one of the MAC contractors administering the demonstration from September 2012 through June 2016.

percent in the first 6 months after implementation (December 2014 through May 2015) to 66 percent in the most recent 6 months for which data are available (October 2016 through March 2017). Some MAC officials attributed this rise in part to provider and supplier education, which improved documentation being submitted.

Table 1. Number of Initial and Resubmission Approval and Denial Decisions for Each Demonstration from Implementation through March 2017

Demonstration	Time period	Initial submissions		Resubmissions	
		Avg. per month	Total requests	Avg. per month	Total requests
Power mobility device	Sep 2012 - Mar 2017	1,861	102,341	628	34,543
Repetitive scheduled non-emergency ambulance services	Dec 2014 - Mar 2017	1,200	33,588	579	16,203
Non-emergency hyperbaric oxygen therapy	Mar 2015 - Mar 2017	105	2,620	24	611
Home health services	Aug 2016 - Mar 2017	15,767	126,132	2,703	21,623
Total			264,681		72,980

Source: GAO analysis of Centers for Medicare & Medicaid Services data. | GAO-18-341.

Notes: Numbers of decisions do not include 34,976 rejected submissions for all demonstrations. Numbers of decisions for power mobility device demonstration do not include decisions made by one of the MAC contractors administering the demonstration from September 2012 through June 2016.

MEDICARE EXPENDITURES DECREASED AFTER PRIOR AUTHORIZATION BEGAN IN FOUR DEMONSTRATIONS

Expenditures Decreased after Prior Authorization Began and Estimated Savings May be as High as About $1.1 to $1.9 Billion, with Most Occurring Soon after Implementation

According to our analysis, expenditures decreased for items and services subject to prior authorization in four demonstrations. For example, expenditure decreases in initial demonstration states from implementation through March 2017 ranged from 17 percent to 74 percent. Figure 3 shows the average monthly expenditures per state from 6 months prior to the start of each demonstration through March 2017 for each of three groups of states: states that were part of the initial demonstration, states that were part of the demonstration expansion, and non-demonstration states. (See app. II for monthly expenditures for items and services covered under each demonstration from their implementation through March 2017).

Our analysis also shows potential savings for items and services subject to prior authorization, based on the difference between actual expenditures and estimates of what expenditures would have been in the absence of the demonstrations. For each demonstration, we estimated expenditures had the demonstration not been implemented by assuming that expenditures would have remained at their average for the 6 months prior to the demonstration starting in each state. We then compared actual expenditures to these estimated expenditures and found that potential savings could be as high as about $1.1 to $1.9 billion.[134]

- Estimated potential savings in states that were part of the demonstrations since either their initial implementation or expansion may be as high as $1.1 billion. For items and services subject to prior authorization in these states, estimated expenditures in the absence of the demonstrations would have been over $2.1 billion, while actual expenditures were about $1.0 billion.

---

[134] CMS has also estimated savings for the demonstrations. However, these estimated savings are not comparable to GAO's estimates because they do not cover the same period of time. For example, CMS's most recent savings estimate for the non-emergency hyperbaric oxygen therapy demonstration is $5.3 million from March 2015 through March 2016.

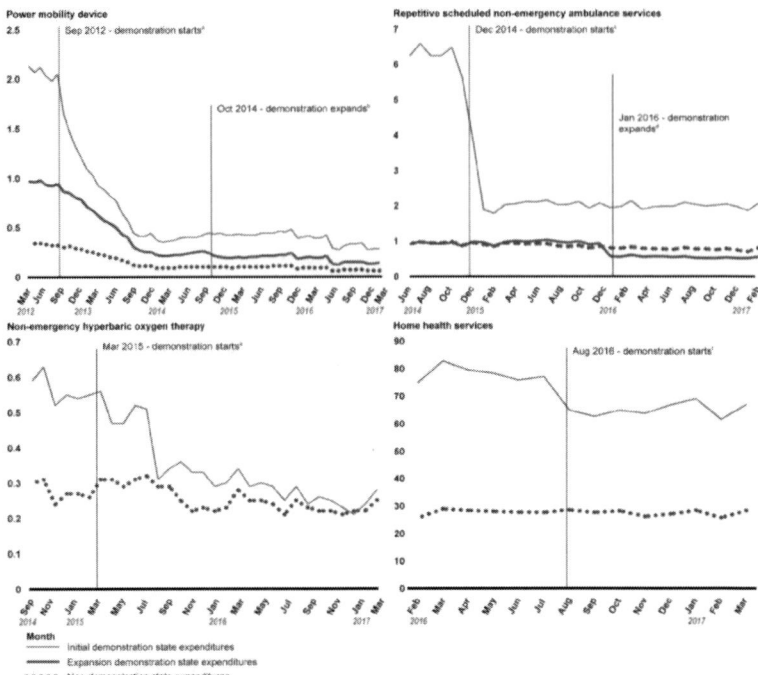

Source: GAO analysis of Centers for Medicare & Medicaid Services data. | GAO-18-341.

Notes: This analysis includes the 50 states and the District of Columbia. The total number of non-demonstration states in each demonstration is: 32 in the power mobility device demonstration, 42 in the repetitive scheduled non-emergency ambulance services demonstration, 48 in the non-emergency hyperbaric oxygen therapy demonstration, and 50 in the home health services demonstration.

[a]Demonstration initially implemented in September 2012 in 7 states: California, Florida, Illinois, Michigan, New York, North Carolina, and Texas.

[b]Demonstration expanded in October 2014 to 12 additional states: Arizona, Georgia, Indiana, Kentucky, Louisiana, Maryland, Missouri, New Jersey, Ohio, Pennsylvania, Tennessee, and Washington.

[c]Demonstration initially implemented in December 2014 in 3 states: New Jersey, Pennsylvania, and South Carolina.

[d]Demonstration expanded in January 2016 to 6 additional states: Delaware, District of Columbia, Maryland, North Carolina, Virginia, and West Virginia.

[e]Demonstration implemented in March 2015 in 3 states: Illinois, Michigan, and New Jersey.

[f]Demonstration implemented in August 2016 in 1 state: Illinois.

Figure 3. Average Monthly Expenditures per State for Four Prior Authorization Demonstrations in Initial Demonstration States, Expansion Demonstration States, and Non-Demonstration States from Six Months Prior to Initial Implementation through March 2017 (in millions).

- Estimated potential savings may be as high as about $1.9 billion if, for the power mobility device demonstration, we estimate savings in both demonstration states and non-demonstration states since implementation. With this method, estimated savings since the power mobility device demonstration's implementation change from over $600 million in demonstration states since each state's implementation to about $1.4 billion in all states since the demonstration began in September 2012, a nearly $800 million increase. This increase is due to including non-demonstration states in the analysis and changing the assumptions for expanded demonstration states in the analysis.[135] CMS officials have reported that certain power mobility device expenditures have declined significantly in both demonstration states and non-demonstration states in part because they think that larger nationwide suppliers improved their compliance with CMS policies in all states based on their experiences with prior authorization. CMS did not make a similar statement for the other demonstrations, and in December 2017, CMS officials said that the agency has not analyzed expenditures in non-demonstration states for the other demonstrations. See Table 2 for estimated potential savings for prior authorization demonstrations from implementation through March 2017.

According to our analysis, more than half of the reduction in monthly expenditures took place within the first 6 months of each demonstration. We calculated the average monthly expenditures for the 6 months prior to the start of each demonstration, the monthly expenditures in the 6th month after implementation, and the monthly expenditures in March 2017 for initial demonstration states in the power mobility device, repetitive

---

[135] Of the nearly $800 million increase in estimated savings, about $370 million of the increase is due to including estimated savings in non-demonstration states from September 2012 through March 2017. The remainder of the increase is due to calculating estimated savings in demonstration expansion states beginning in September 2012 (demonstration implementation) instead of October 2014 (demonstration expansion) and calculating the average expenditures for the 6 months prior to the demonstration starting in September 2012 instead of 6 months prior to the demonstration expanding in October 2014.

scheduled non-emergency ambulance services, and non-emergency hyperbaric oxygen therapy demonstrations. We compared these expenditures and found that 58, 99, and 91 percent of the reduction in monthly expenditures during this time took place during the first 6 months of each demonstration, respectively.[136]

Table 2. Estimated Potential Savings for Prior Authorization in Four Demonstrations from Implementation through March 2017

	Estimated potential savings in demonstration states[a]	
	Group of states (number of states)	Estimated savings (in millions)
Repetitive scheduled non-emergency ambulance services	Initial demonstration states (3)	$349.5
	Expansion demonstration states (6)	38.0
Non-emergency hyperbaric oxygen therapy	Initial demonstration states (3)	17.6
Home health services	Initial demonstration state (1)	104.2
Power mobility device	Initial demonstration states (7)	590.1
	Expansion demonstration states (12)	17.8
Total estimated savings		1,117.2
Additional estimated potential savings for power mobility device demonstration in expansion and non-demonstration states[b]		
Power mobility device	Expansion demonstration states (12)[c]	411.1
	Non-demonstration states (32)[c]	367.5
	Total estimated savings, including additional estimated savings for power mobility device demonstration	1,895.8

Source: GAO analysis of Centers for Medicare & Medicaid Services data. | GAO-18-341.

[a]Estimated potential savings in states that were part of the demonstrations since either their initial implementation or expansion, assuming that total expenditures would have remained at their average for the 6 months prior to the demonstration starting in each state.

[b]Because CMS stated that the power mobility device demonstration may result in savings in all states—even those not part of the demonstration—we also estimated potential savings for that demonstration in non-demonstration states.

[c]Additional estimated potential savings in expansion demonstration states is due to calculating estimated savings in demonstration expansion states beginning in September 2012 (demonstration implementation) instead of October 2014 (demonstration expansion) and calculating the average expenditures for the 6 months prior to the demonstration starting in September 2012 instead of 6 months prior to the demonstration expanding in October 2014.

---

[136] For purposes of this analysis, we excluded the home health services demonstration because it was in effect for only 8 months before it was put on pause in April 2017. As of February 2018, the demonstration has not resumed.

Other CMS Efforts May Have Contributed to Expenditure Reductions

CMS had other program integrity efforts underway before implementing prior authorization, and these efforts may have also contributed to the reduction in expenditures for items and services subject to prior authorization in these demonstrations. CMS officials said that it is likely that prior authorization played a large role in the expenditure reduction for those select items and services. However, CMS officials also reported that it is difficult to separate the effects of prior authorization from other program integrity efforts, and the agency has not developed a methodology for determining the independent effect of prior authorization on expenditures. We found that some of these other program integrity efforts have addressed provider screening and enrollment and certain durable medical equipment, and these may have contributed to the reductions in Medicare expenditures.[137]

Provider Screening and Enrollment

CMS has taken steps to keep potentially fraudulent providers and suppliers from billing Medicare. For example,

- in September 2011, CMS began revalidating providers' and suppliers' enrollment in Medicare to ensure that they continue to be eligible to bill Medicare. Revalidation involves confirming that the provider or supplier continues to meet Medicaid program requirements, including ensuring that a provider or supplier does not employ or contract with individuals who have been excluded from participation in federal health care programs.[138] We previously reported that screening all providers and suppliers—not just the ones subject to prior authorization—resulted in over

---

[137] We recently reported on some of these efforts as steps CMS has taken to target high-risk areas within the Medicare program. See GAO *Medicare and Medicaid: CMS Needs to Fully Align Its Efforts with Fraud Risk Framework*, GAO-18-88 (Washington, D.C.: December 2017).
[138] 42 CFR 424.515.

23,000 new applications being denied or rejected and over 703,000 existing enrollment records being deactivated or revoked from March 2011 through December 2015.[139] We also reported that CMS estimated the revised process avoided $2.4 billion in total Medicare payments to ineligible providers and suppliers from March 2011 to May 2015, some of which may have been payments for items and services subject to prior authorization.

- in July 2013, CMS implemented moratoria on enrollment of new providers for home health services and for repetitive, scheduled non-emergency ambulance transport in select counties. As of January 2018, CMS had extended the home health services moratoria statewide to Florida, Illinois, Michigan, and Texas and the repetitive, scheduled non-emergency ambulance transport moratoria statewide to Pennsylvania and New Jersey. During a moratorium, no new applications to enroll as a billing provider of the affected service types are reviewed or approved.[140] In October 2017, CMS officials said that home health and non-emergency ambulance services' expenditures may have been affected by provider enrollment moratoria.

Certain Durable Medical Equipment Pricing, Payments, and Education and Outreach

CMS has taken steps to change how certain durable medical equipment is paid for and to provide ongoing durable medical equipment education and outreach. For example,

- in January 2011, CMS implemented a DMEPOS competitive bidding program required by the Medicare Prescription Drug,

---

[139] See GAO, *Medicare: Initial Results of Revised Process to Screen Providers and Suppliers, and Need for Objectives and Performance Measures*, GAO-17-42 (Washington, D.C.: November 2016).

[140] CMS may impose temporary moratoria on a particular provider or supplier type or a particular geographic area as a program integrity effort to prevent fraud, waste, and abuse. See 42 U.S.C. § 1395cc(j)(7).

Improvement, and Modernization Act of 2003.[141] Under the program, only competitively selected contract suppliers can furnish certain durable medical equipment items at competitively determined prices to Medicare beneficiaries in designated areas. CMS began the program in 9 of the largest metropolitan areas, and in July 2013 expanded to an additional 100 large metropolitan areas.[142] In January 2016, CMS implemented competitive bidding program-based adjusted prices for non-designated areas for durable medical equipment items that were previously, or are currently, included in the competitive bidding program. According to CMS, the program—which generally results in lower competitively bid prices—is reducing expenditures for approximately half of the beneficiaries receiving power mobility devices nationwide. We have previously reported that prices decreased for power mobility devices in the competitive bidding program; some of these devices are also subject to prior authorization.[143]

- in January 2011, CMS eliminated the lump sum purchase option for standard power wheelchairs. This change reduced expenditures for power wheelchairs used on a short-term basis because payments for short-term rentals are lower than for the purchase of these items.
- durable medical equipment MACs and CMS provide continuous DMEPOS education and outreach. According to CMS, the education and outreach may have contributed to reducing expenditures for power mobility devices by helping providers and suppliers to understand how to bill correctly and to submit fewer claims that do not meet Medicare coverage and payment requirements.

---

[141] Pub. L. No. 108-173, § 302(b), 117 Stat. 2066, 2224 (2003) (codified at 42 U.S.C. § 1395w-3).

[142] The metropolitan areas are metropolitan statistical areas or a part thereof. Metropolitan statistical areas are designated by the Office of Management and Budget and include major cities and the suburban areas surrounding them.

[143] See GAO, *Medicare: Bidding Results from CMS's Durable Medical Equipment Competitive Bidding Program*, GAO-15-63 (Washington, D.C.: November 2014).

Providers and Suppliers Reported that Prior Authorization Is an Effective Tool, but They Face Difficulty Obtaining Documentation, and Concerns Exist for One Program

Many Providers and Suppliers Reported Prior Authorization Benefits, and CMS Has Addressed Some of Their Initial Concerns

Many of the officials we interviewed representing provider, supplier, and beneficiary groups, as well as CMS and MACs, reported benefits to prior authorization. Officials from some of these groups said that prior authorization is an effective tool to reduce unnecessary utilization and improper payments. Some officials who reported benefits said that prior authorization helps educate providers and suppliers about allowable items and services under Medicare and improves providers' and suppliers' documentation. Some officials also said that providers and suppliers appreciate the assurance of knowing that Medicare is likely to pay for these items and services. Officials from three provider and supplier groups said that by getting provisional prior authorization, their claims will likely not be denied, and they can thus avoid the appeals process, for which there are significant delays.[144] In addition, officials from two provider and supplier groups believe that prior authorization may deter fraudulent suppliers from participating in Medicare. Because of these benefits, these provider and supplier group officials recommended that CMS expand its use of prior authorization.

---

[144] See GAO, *Medicare Fee-For-Service: Opportunities Remain to Improve Appeals Process*, GAO-16-366 (Washington, D.C.: May 2016).

In addition, CMS has improved the prior authorization programs by responding to some of the providers' and suppliers' initial concerns. For example, for the power mobility device demonstration, CMS and MAC officials that process DMEPOS claims reported that providers and suppliers were initially confused about whether beneficiaries with representative payees—persons or organizations authorized to accept payment on a beneficiary's behalf—were exempt from the prior authorization program.[145] To address this issue, CMS revised and clarified its guidance related to representative payees. In addition, for the non-emergency hyperbaric oxygen therapy demonstration, officials from CMS and a MAC administering the demonstration said that providers and suppliers raised concerns that a Medicare-covered condition (compromised skin grafts) included in the demonstration required immediate care and therefore should not be subject to prior authorization. In response, CMS removed the condition from the list of conditions subject to prior authorization.

Providers and Suppliers Report Difficulty Obtaining Documentation for Prior Authorization Requests, and CMS Is Taking Steps to Address This Challenge

Some provider and supplier group officials we interviewed reported that obtaining the documentation necessary to submit a prior authorization request can be difficult. For example, some of these officials told us that providers and suppliers may spend 3 to 7 weeks obtaining necessary documentation from referring physicians and other relevant parties before submitting a prior authorization request. While CMS's documentation requirements did not change under prior authorization, officials from a provider and supplier group we spoke with said that prior authorization exacerbates existing documentation challenges because they must obtain all required documentation before providing items and services to

---

[145] Beneficiaries may require a representative payee if they are deemed incapable of managing their finances, for example, due to a cognitive impairment.

beneficiaries. As we noted in a previous report, two durable medical equipment MACs said that referring physicians may lack financial incentives to submit proper documentation since they are unaffected if a durable medical equipment or home health claim is denied due to insufficient documentation, while the provider or supplier submitting the claim loses the payment.[146]

Furthermore, according to some provider and supplier group representatives, CMS's documentation requirements can be difficult to meet. Representatives from one supplier and provider group said that there is a high standard of proof to meet the information needed to support their medical necessity requirements. For example, documentation in the medical record is required to show whether the referring physician considered other options. Also, representatives from another provider and suppler group said that, unlike private insurers, CMS has more requirements that providers and suppliers consider administrative. For instance, MACs deny prior authorization requests for missing physician signatures.

In addition, representatives from a provider and supplier group said it may be necessary to collect documentation from multiple providers that treated the beneficiary in order to meet CMS's medical necessity requirements. However, officials from one private insurer said that their medical necessity requirements for certain items and services may necessitate receiving documentation from several providers as well, although this does not occur often.

CMS officials acknowledged that the agency's requirements may be more difficult to meet than those of private health insurers. However, this scrutiny may be beneficial because, unlike private insurers, Medicare must pay for health care delivered by any eligible physician willing to accept Medicare payment and follow Medicare requirements.

---

[146] See GAO, *Medicare Provider Education: Oversight of Efforts to Reduce Improper Billing Needs Improvement*, GAO-17-290 (Washington, D.C.: March 2017).

We found that CMS and the MACs have taken some steps to assist providers and suppliers in obtaining documentation from referring physicians. For example, CMS has created e-clinical templates for home health services and power mobility devices that can be incorporated into progress notes to help ensure physicians meet medical necessity requirements. CMS and the MACs have also created documentation checklists, prior authorization coversheets, and other tools to assist providers and suppliers in verifying that they have obtained the documentation necessary to meet CMS's documentation requirements. Agency officials have stated that they are working on additional changes to reduce provider and supplier burden, for example, developing e-clinical templates for additional items and services.

Furthermore, representatives from each of the MACs said that they call providers and suppliers that receive certain prior authorization non-affirmations to ensure suppliers and providers understand what information is required to obtain a provisional affirmation.[147] Some MAC representatives said that having a phone conversation with suppliers allows them to resolve non-affirmations more expediently and reduces the number of resubmissions. Representatives from one MAC estimated that when they call providers and suppliers, they are able to resolve 50 to 80 percent of the issues that led to the non-affirmations. Several MAC representatives also said calling helps providers and suppliers gain a better understanding of CMS's documentation requirements, which will increase their likelihood of having future requests provisionally affirmed. In addition, CMS officials said that the agency encourages MACs to call referring physicians directly, when necessary, to remedy curable errors or obtain additional documentation needed to affirm a request because non-affirmation may be resolved faster without providers and suppliers serving as intermediaries.[148]

---

[147] CMS requires the MACs to call providers and suppliers participating in the home health demonstration and the permanent DMEPOS program. The MACs that administer the other demonstrations call as a best practice.

[148] CMS officials said that, for example, a curable error for the home health pre-claim review would be when the medical record supports that the person is homebound and needs skilled services, but the documentation for the face-to-face examination between the person and referring physician is missing or has not been signed by the referring physician.

Providers and Suppliers Report Concerns about Whether the Permanent DMEPOS Program Includes Essential Accessories

Providers and suppliers reported concerns about whether accessories deemed essential to group 3 power wheelchairs are subject to prior authorization and can be provisionally affirmed under the permanent DMEPOS program. According to CMS, the permanent DMEPOS program requires prior authorization for power wheelchair bases, but not for their accessories. CMS officials said this is because accessories do not meet the criteria for inclusion on the Master List. However, according to CMS, the MACs must review these accessories when they make prior authorization determinations because their decision to provisionally affirm a wheelchair base is based in part on their view of the medical necessity of the accessories. Therefore, if an essential accessory does not meet medical necessity requirements, a MAC will deny a prior authorization request for a power wheelchair base. In other words, in practice these accessories are subject to prior authorization, even though they are not technically included in the permanent DMEPOS program and therefore cannot be provisionally affirmed. As a result, providers and suppliers lack assurance about whether Medicare is likely to pay for these accessories.

In December 2017, CMS officials stated that there have been preliminary discussions regarding the feasibility and effect of subjecting accessories essential to the group 3 power wheelchairs in the permanent DMEPOS program to prior authorization. However, CMS officials did not provide a timeframe for reaching a decision about whether they would do so. Federal internal control standards state that agencies should design control activities that enable an agency to achieve its objectives and should respond to any risks related to achieving those objectives.[149] By not including essential accessories in prior authorization so they can be provisionally affirmed as appropriate, CMS may hinder its ability to achieve one of the stated benefits of the prior authorization program—to

---

[149] See GAO-14-704G.

allow providers and suppliers to know prior to providing the items whether Medicare will likely pay for them.

CMS MONITORS PRIOR AUTHORIZATION BUT HAS NOT MADE PLANS FOR PRIOR AUTHORIZATION IN THE FUTURE

CMS Monitors Prior Authorization and Has Contracted for Evaluations of the Demonstrations

We found that CMS monitoring includes reviewing MAC reports of the results of prior authorization requests, examining MAC timeliness and accuracy, and contracting for independent evaluations of the prior authorization demonstrations.

- CMS officials told us that they review weekly, monthly, and annual MAC reports that include information such as numbers of requests received, completed, approved, denied, and resubmitted.
- According to CMS officials, they monitor MAC timeliness through these reports and separately have a contractor review MAC accuracy in processing requests. According to these officials, they have not identified any issues with MAC timeliness, as the MACs currently meet the standards for processing initial requests within 10 business days and resubmissions within 20 business days. In addition, CMS officials said that a sample of MACs' prior authorization decisions is reviewed each month for accuracy for each of the prior authorization demonstrations, and the reviews have not identified any issues with these decisions.
- CMS officials said that they meet with providers and supplier groups regularly to solicit feedback, to identify issues that need to be addressed, and to determine whether there are any problems, such as reduced beneficiary access to care. According to CMS

officials, they have not identified any negative impact on beneficiary access to care as a result of implementing prior authorization.

- CMS has contracted for independent evaluations of the power mobility device, repetitive scheduled non-emergency ambulance services, and non-emergency hyperbaric oxygen demonstrations. In December 2017, CMS officials told us that evaluations will be completed and results available after the demonstrations end.[150] In December 2017, officials told us that they also plan to contract for an evaluation of the permanent program after more time has passed.

Although Most Prior Authorization Is Scheduled to End in 2018, CMS Does Not Have Plans to Continue Efforts

Most prior authorization programs are scheduled to end in 2018, with all the demonstrations concluding and only the limited permanent program remaining.

- The non-emergency hyperbaric oxygen demonstration ended in February 2018, the power mobility device demonstration in August 2018, and the repetitive scheduled non-emergency ambulance services demonstration in November 2018.
- The home health services demonstration has been on pause since April 2017 with no plans to resume as of February 2018, although CMS stated that they are considering improvements to the demonstration.

---

[150] For the power mobility device and repetitive scheduled non-emergency ambulance demonstrations, CMS officials provided us interim reports of the independent evaluations. An interim report of the non-emergency hyperbaric oxygen therapy demonstration was not available at the time of our review. In August 2017 CMS officials told us that they had not contracted for an evaluation of the home health services demonstration because it had been paused.

- The permanent program, which currently consists of two group 3 power wheelchairs, is the only prior authorization program that will remain. According to CMS officials, these wheelchairs are very low volume, and the HHS Office of the Inspector General reported that these wheelchairs represent just a small percentage of all durable medical equipment claims.[151]

CMS has not made plans for continuing expiring or paused prior authorization programs or expanding prior authorization. However, officials told us that they would like to see prior authorization for additional items. For example, CMS officials said that they have considered prior authorization for items such as hospital beds and oxygen concentrators, because these have high utilization or improper payment rates. In addition, in December 2017, CMS officials said that the agency is evaluating whether it has met the requirements for nationwide expansion of the repetitive scheduled non-emergency ambulance services demonstration established by the Medicare Access and CHIP Reauthorization Act of 2015. However, CMS officials also said that have not yet determined the next steps for the use of prior authorization. Federal internal control standards state that agencies should identify, analyze, and respond to risks related to achieving objectives.[152] By not taking steps, based on results from the evaluations, to continue prior authorization, CMS risks missed opportunities for achieving its stated goals of reducing costs and realizing program savings by reducing unnecessary utilization and improper payments.

---

[151] See HHS Office of the Inspector General, Medicare Power Wheelchair Claims Frequently Did Not Meet Documentation Requirements, OEI-04-07-00401 (Washington, D.C.: December 2009).
[152] See GAO-14-704G.

Conclusion

Since September 2012, CMS has begun using prior authorization to ensure that Medicare coverage and payment rules have been met before the agency pays for selected items and services. During this time, expenditures for items and services subject to prior authorization have been reduced. We estimate potential savings may be as high as about $1.1 to $1.9 billion, although other CMS program integrity efforts may have contributed to these reductions. Many stakeholders, including providers, suppliers, and MAC officials, support prior authorization, citing benefits such as reduced unnecessary utilization. However, providers and suppliers report concerns about whether accessories deemed essential to group 3 power wheelchairs are subject to prior authorization and can be provisionally affirmed. By not including essential accessories in prior authorization, CMS may hinder its ability to achieve one of the stated benefits of the prior authorization program—to allow providers and suppliers to know prior to providing the items whether Medicare will likely pay for them.

All four prior authorization demonstrations are either paused or will end in 2018, and CMS does not have plans to extend these programs or expand the use of prior authorization to additional items and services with high rates of unnecessary utilization or improper payments. By not taking steps, based on results from the evaluations, to continue prior authorization, CMS risks missed opportunities for achieving its stated goals of reducing costs and realizing program savings by reducing unnecessary utilization and improper payments.

Recommendations for Executive Action

We are making the following two recommendations to CMS.

- The Administrator of CMS should subject accessories essential to the group 3 power wheelchairs in the permanent DMEPOS program to prior authorization. (Recommendation 1)
- The Administrator of CMS should take steps, based on results from evaluations, to continue prior authorization. These steps could include:
  - resuming the paused home health services demonstration;
  - extending current demonstrations; or,
  - identifying new opportunities for expanding prior authorization to additional items and services with high unnecessary utilization and high improper payment rates. (Recommendation 2).

AGENCY COMMENTS

We provided a draft of this report to HHS for comment, and its comments are reprinted in appendix III. HHS also provided technical comments, which we incorporated as appropriate.

HHS neither agreed nor disagreed with the recommendations but said it would continue to evaluate prior authorization programs and take our findings and recommendations into consideration in developing plans or determining appropriate next steps. In addition, in response to our recommendation to take steps to continue prior authorization, HHS noted that the President's fiscal year 2019 budget for HHS included a legislative proposal to extend its statutory authority to permanently require prior authorization for specified Medicare fee-for-service items and services to all Medicare fee-for-service items and services.

As agreed with your office, unless you publicly announce the contents of this report earlier, we plan no further distribution until 30 days from the report date. At that time, we will send copies to the Secretary of Health and Human Services, the Administrator of the Centers for Medicare &

Medicaid Services, and other interested parties. In addition, the report is available at no charge on the GAO website at http://www.gao.gov.

If you or your staff have any questions about this report, please contact A. Nicole Clowers at (202) 512-7114 or clowersa@gao.gov or Kathleen M. King at (202) 512-7114 or kingk@gao.gov. Contact points for our Offices of Congressional Relations and Public Affairs may be found on the last page of this report. Major contributors to this report are listed in appendix IV.

Sincerely yours,
A. Nicole Clowers
Managing Director, Health Care
Kathleen M. King
Director, Health Care

APPENDIX I: LIST OF ITEMS THAT MAY BE SELECTED FOR PRIOR AUTHORIZATION

In December 2015, the Centers for Medicare & Medicaid Services (CMS) established a permanent prior authorization program for certain durable medical equipment, prosthetics, orthotics, and supplies (DMEPOS).[1] To select the items subject to prior authorization, CMS compiled a Master List of items that 1) appear on the DMEPOS Fee Schedule list, 2) have an average purchase fee of $1,000 or greater (adjusted annually for inflation) or an average rental fee schedule of $100 or greater (adjusted annually for inflation), and 3) meet one of these two criteria: the item was identified in a GAO or Department of Health and Human Services Office of Inspector General report that is national in scope and published in 2007 or later as having a high rate of fraud or unnecessary utilization, or the item is listed in the 2011 or later published Comprehensive Error Rate Testing program's annual report.[2] The information presented in this appendix was reprinted from information in a

December 2015 final rule. We did not edit it in any way, such as to spell out abbreviations. (See Table 3 for the Master List.)

Table 3. Master List of Durable Medical Equipment, Prosthetics, Orthotics, and Supplies Subject to Frequent Unnecessary Utilization for Prior Authorization

Healthcare Common Procedure Coding System Code	Item Description
E0193	Powered air flotation bed (low air loss therapy).
E0260	Hosp bed semi-electr w/matt.
E0277	Powered pres-redu air mattrs.
E0371	Non-powered advanced pressure reducing overlay for mattress, standard mattress length and width.
E0372	Powered air overlay for mattress, standard mattress length and width.
E0373	Non-powered advanced pressure reducing mattress.
E0470	Respiratory assist device, bi-level pressure capability, without backup rate feature, used with noninvasive interface, e.g., nasal or facial mask (intermittent assist device with continuous positive airway pressure device)
E0601	Continuous Airway Pressure (CPAP) Device.
E1390	Oxygen Concentrator.
E2402	Negative pressure wound therapy electrical pump, stationary or portable.
K0004	High strength, lightweight wheelchair.
K0813	Power wheelchair, group 1 standard, portable, sling/solid seat and back, patient weight capacity up to and including 300 pounds.
K0814	Power wheelchair, group 1 standard, portable, captains chair, patient weight capacity up to and including 300pounds.
K0815	Power wheelchair, group 1 standard, sling/solid seat and back, patient weight capacity up to and including 300 pounds.
K0816	Power wheelchair, group 1 standard, captains chair, patient weight capacity up to and including 300 pounds.
K0820	Power wheelchair, group 2 standard, portable, sling/solid seat/back, patient weight capacity up to and including 300 pounds.
K0821	Power wheelchair, group 2 standard, portable, captains chair, patient weight capacity up to and including 300pounds.
K0822	Power wheelchair, group 2 standard, sling/solid seat/back, patient weight capacity up to and including 300 pounds.
K0823	Power wheelchair, group 2 standard, captains chair, patient weight capacity up to and including 300 pounds.
K0824	Power wheelchair, group 2 heavy duty, sling/solid seat/back, patient weight capacity 301 to 450 pounds.

Table 3. (Continued)

Healthcare Common Procedure Coding System Code	Item Description
K0825	Power wheelchair, group 2 heavy duty, captains chair, patient weight capacity 301 to 450 pounds.
K0826	Power wheelchair, group 2 very heavy duty, sling/solid seat/back, patient weight capacity 451 to 600 pounds.
K0827	Power wheelchair, group 2 very heavy duty, captains chair, patient weight capacity 451 to 600 pounds.
K0828	Power wheelchair, group 2 extra heavy duty, sling/solid seat/back, patient weight capacity 601 pounds or more.
K0829	Power wheelchair, group 2 extra heavy duty, captains chair, patient weight 601 pounds or more.
K0835	Power wheelchair, group 2 standard, single power option, sling/solid seat/back, patient weight capacity up to and including 300 pound
K0836	Power wheelchair, group 2 standard, single power option, captains chair, patient weight capacity up to and including 300 pounds.
K0837	Power wheelchair, group 2 heavy duty, single power option, sling/solid seat/back, patient weight capacity 301to 450 pounds.
K0838	Power wheelchair, group 2 heavy duty, single power option, captains chair, patient weight capacity 301 to 450 pounds.
K0839	Power wheelchair, group 2 very heavy duty, single power option sling/solid seat/back, patient weight capacity451 to 600 pounds.
K0840	Power wheelchair, group 2 extra heavy duty, single power option, sling/solid seat/back, patient weight capacity 601 pounds or more.
K0841	Power wheelchair, group 2 standard, multiple power option, sling/solid seat/back, patient weight capacity up to and including 300 pounds
K0842	Power wheelchair, group 2 standard, multiple power option, captains chair, patient weight capacity up to and including 300 pounds.
K0843	Power wheelchair, group 2 heavy duty, multiple power option, sling/solid seat/back, patient weight capacity 301 to 450 pounds.
K0848	Power wheelchair, group 3 standard, sling/solid seat/back, patient weight capacity up to and including 300 pounds.
K0849	Power wheelchair, group 3 standard, captains chair, patient weight capacity up to and including 300 pounds.
K0850	Power wheelchair, group 3 heavy duty, sling/solid seat/back, patient weight capacity 301 to 450 pounds.
K0851	Power wheelchair, group 3 heavy duty, captains chair, patient weight capacity 301 to 450 pounds.
K0852	Power wheelchair, group 3 very heavy duty, sling/solid seat/back, patient weight capacity 451 to 600 pounds.
K0853	Power wheelchair, group 3 very heavyduty, captains chair, patient weight capacity 451 to 600 pounds.

Medicare

Healthcare Common Procedure Coding System Code	Item Description
K0854	Power wheelchair, group 3 extra heavy duty, sling/solid seat/back, patient weight capacity 601 pounds or more.
K0855	Power wheelchair, group 3 extra heavy duty, captains chair, patient weight capacity 601 pounds or more.
K0856	Power wheelchair, group 3 standard, single power option, sling/solid seat/back, patient weight capacity up to and including 300 pound
K0857	Power wheelchair, group 3 standard, single power option, captains chair, patient weight capacity up to and including 300 pounds.
K0858	Power wheelchair, group 3 heavy duty, single power option, sling/solid seat/back, patient weight 301 to 450 pounds.
K0859	Power wheelchair, group 3 heavy duty, single power option, captains chair, patient weight capacity 301 to 450 pounds
K0860	Power wheelchair, group 3 very heavy duty, single power option, sling/solid seat/back, patient weight capacity 451 to 600 pounds.
K0861	Power wheelchair, group 3 standard, multiple power option, sling/solid seat/back, patient weight capacity up to and including 300 pounds
K0862	Power wheelchair, group 3 heavy duty, multiple power option, sling/solid seat/back, patient weight capacity 301 to 450 pounds.
K0863	Power wheelchair, group 3 very heavy duty, multiple power option, sling/solid seat/back, patient weight capacity 451 to 600 pounds.
K0864	Power wheelchair, group 3 extra heavy duty, multiple power option, sling/solid seat/back, patient weight capacity 601 pounds or more.
L5010	Partial foot, molded socket, ankle height, with toe filler.
L5020	Partial foot, molded socket, tibial tubercle height, with toe filler.
L5050	Ankle, symes, molded socket, sach foot.
L5060	Ankle, symes, metal frame, molded leather socket, articulated ankle/foot.
L5100	Below knee, molded socket, shin, sach foot.
L5105	Below knee, plastic socket, joints and thigh lacer, sach foot.
L5150	Knee disarticulation (or through knee), molded socket, external knee joints, shin, sach foot.
L5160	Knee disarticulation (or through knee), molded socket, bent knee configuration, external knee joints, shin, sach foot.
L5200	Above knee, molded socket, single axis constant friction knee, shin, sach foot.
L5210	Above knee, short prosthesis, no knee joint('stubbies'), with foot blocks, no ankle joints, each.
L5220	Above knee, short prosthesis, no knee joint ('stubbies'), with articulated ankle/foot, dynamically aligned, each.
L5230	Above knee, for proximal femoral focal deficiency, constant friction knee, shin, sach foot.
L5250	Hip disarticulation, canadian type; molded socket, hip joint, single axis constant friction knee, shin, sach foot.

Table 3. (Continued)

Healthcare Common Procedure Coding System Code	Item Description
L5270	Hip disarticulation, tilt table type; molded socket, locking hip joint, single axis constant friction knee, shin, sach foot.
L5280	Hemipelvectomy, canadian type; molded socket, hip joint, single axis constant friction knee, shin, sach foot.
L5301	Below knee, molded socket, shin, sach foot, endoskeletal system.
L5312	Knee disarticulation (or through knee), molded socket, single axis knee, pylon, sach foot, endoskeletal system.
L5321	Above knee, molded socket, open end, sach foot, endoskeletal system, single axis knee.
L5331	Hip disarticulation, canadian type, molded socket, endoskeletal system, hip joint, single axis knee, sach foot.
L5341	Hemipelvectomy, canadian type, molded socket, endoskeletal system, hip joint, single axis knee, sach foot.
L5400	Immediate post surgicalor early fitting, application of initial rigid dressing, including fitting, alignment, suspension, and one cast change, below knee
L5420	Immediate post surgical or early fitting, application of initial rigid dressing, including fitting, alignment and suspension and one cast change 'ak'or knee disarticulation
L5500	Initial, below knee 'ptb'type socket, non-alignable system, pylon, no cover, sach foot, plaster socket, direct formed.
L5505	Initial, above knee—knee disarticulation, ischial level socket, non-alignable system, pylon, no cover, sach foot, plaster socket, direct formed
L5510	Preparatory, below knee 'ptb'type socket, non-alignable system, pylon, no cover, sach foot, plaster socket, molded to model.
L5520	Preparatory, below knee 'ptb'type socket, non-alignable system, pylon, no cover, sach foot, thermoplastic orequal, direct formed.
L5530	Preparatory, below knee 'ptb'type socket, non-alignable system, pylon, no cover, sach foot, thermoplastic orequal, molded to model.
L5535	Preparatory,below knee 'ptb'type socket, non-alignable system, no cover, sach foot, prefabricated, adjustable open end socket.
L5540	Preparatory, below knee 'ptb'type socket, non-alignable system, pylon, no cover, sach foot, laminated socket, molded to model.
L5560	Preparatory, above knee—knee disarticulation, ischial level socket, non-alignable system, pylon, no cover, sach foot, plaster socket, molded to model
L5570	Preparatory, above knee—knee disarticulation, ischial level socket, non-alignablesystem, pylon, no cover, sach foot, thermoplastic or equal, direct formed

Medicare

Healthcare Common Procedure Coding System Code	Item Description
L5580	Preparatory, above knee—knee disarticulation ischial level socket, non-alignable system, pylon, no cover, sach foot, thermoplastic or equal, molded to model
L5585	Preparatory, above knee—knee disarticulation, ischial level socket, non-alignable system, pylon, no cover, sach foot, prefabricated adjustable open end socket
L5590	Preparatory, above knee—knee disarticulation ischial level socket, non-alignablesystem, pylon no cover, sach foot, laminated socket, molded to model
L5595	Preparatory, hip disarticulation-hemipelvectomy, pylon, no cover, sach foot, thermoplastic or equal, molded to patient model.
L5600	Preparatory, hip disarticulation-hemipelvectomy, pylon, no cover, sach foot, laminated socket, molded to patient model.
L5610	Addition to lower extremity, endoskeletal system, above knee, hydracadence system.
L5611	Addition to lower extremity, endoskeletalsystem, above knee—knee disarticulation, 4 bar linkage, with friction swing phase control.
L5613	Addition to lower extremity, endoskeletal system, above knee—knee disarticulation, 4 bar linkage, with hydraulic swing phase control.
L5614	Addition to lower extremity, exoskeletal system, above knee—knee disarticulation, 4 bar linkage, with pneumatic swing phase control.
L5616	Addition to lower extremity, endoskeletal system, above knee, universal multiplex system, friction swing phase control.
L5639	Addition to lower extremity, below knee, wood socket.
L5643	Addition to lower extremity, hip disarticulation, flexible inner socket, external frame.
L5649	Addition to lower extremity, ischial containment/narrow m-l socket.
L5651	Addition to lower extremity, above knee, flexible inner socket, external frame.
L5681	Addition to lower extremity, below knee/above knee, custom fabricated socket insert for congenital or atypicaltraumatic amputee, silicone gel, elastomeric or equal, for use with or without locking mechanism, initial only (for other than initial, use code l5673 or l5679)
L5683	Addition to lower extremity, below knee/above knee, custom fabricated socket insert for other than congenitalor atypical traumatic amputee, silicone gel, elastomeric or equal, for use with or without locking mechanism, initial only (for other than initial, use code l5673 or l5679)
L5700	Replacement, socket, below knee, molded to patient model.
L5701	Replacement, socket, above knee/knee disarticulation, including attachment plate, molded to patient model.
L5702	Replacement, socket, hip disarticulation, including hip joint, molded to patient model.

Table 3. (Continued)

Healthcare Common Procedure Coding System Code	Item Description
L5703	Ankle, symes, molded to patient model, socket without solid ankle cushion heel (sach) foot, replacement only.
L5707	Customshaped protective cover, hip disarticulation.
L5724	Addition, exoskeletal knee-shin system, single axis, fluid swing phase control.
L5726	Addition, exoskeletal knee-shin system, single axis, external joints fluid swing phase control.
L5728	Addition, exoskeletal knee-shin system, single axis, fluid swing and stance phase control.
L5780	Addition, exoskeletal knee-shin system, single axis, pneumatic/hydra pneumatic swing phase control.
L5781	Addition to lower limb prosthesis, vacuum pump, residual limb volume management and moisture evacuation system.
L5782	Addition to lower limb prosthesis, vacuum pump, residual limb volume management and moisture evacuation system, heavy duty.
L5795	Addition, exoskeletal system, hip disarticulation, ultra-light material (titanium, carbon fiber or equal).
L5814	Addition, endoskeletal knee-shin system, polycentric, hydraulic swing phase control, mechanical stance phase lock.
L5818	Addition, endoskeletal knee-shin system, polycentric, friction swing, and stance phase control.
L5822	Addition, endoskeletal knee-shin system, single axis, pneumatic swing, friction stance phase control.
L5824	Addition, endoskeletal knee-shin system, single axis, fluid swing phase control.
L5826	Addition, endoskeletal knee-shin system, single axis, hydraulic swing phase control, with miniature high activity frame.
L5828	Addition, endoskeletal knee-shin system, single axis, fluid swing and stance phase control.
L5830	Addition, endoskeletal knee-shin system, single axis, pneumatic/swing phase control.
L5840	Addition, endoskeletal knee/shin system, 4-bar linkage or multiaxial, pneumatic swing phase control.
L5845	Addition, endoskeletal, knee-shin system, stance flexion feature, adjustable.
L5848	Addition to endoskeletal knee-shin system, fluid stance extension, dampening feature, with or without adjustability.
L5856	Addition to lower extremity prosthesis, endoskeletal knee-shin system, microprocessor control feature, swing and stance phase, includes electronic sensor(s), any type

Healthcare Common Procedure Coding System Code	Item Description
L5857	Addition to lower extremity prosthesis, endoskeletal knee-shin system, microprocessor control feature, swing phase only, includes electronic sensor(s), any type
L5858	Addition to lower extremity prosthesis, endoskeletal knee shin system, microprocessor control feature, stance phase only, includes electronic sensor(s), any type
L5930	Addition, endoskeletal system, high activity knee control frame.
L5960	Addition, endoskeletalsystem, hip disarticulation, ultra-light material (titanium, carbon fiber or equal).
L5964	Addition, endoskeletal system, above knee, flexible protective outer surface covering system.
L5966	Addition, endoskeletal system, hip disarticulation, flexible protective outer surface covering system.
L5968	Addition to lower limb prosthesis, multiaxial ankle with swing phase active dorsiflexion feature.
L5973	Endoskeletal ankle foot system, microprocessor controlled feature, dorsiflexion and/or plantar flexion control, includes power source
L5979	All lower extremity prosthesis, multi-axial ankle, dynamic response foot, one piece system.
L5980	All lower extremity prostheses, flex foot system.
L5981	All lower extremity prostheses, flex-walk system or equal.
L5987	All lower extremity prosthesis, shank foot system with vertical loading pylon.
L5988	Addition to lower limb prosthesis, vertical shock reducing pylon feature.
L5990	Addition to lower extremity prosthesis, user adjustable heel height.

Source: Medicare Program; Prior Authorization Process for Certain Durable Medical Equipment, Prosthetics, Orthotics, and Supplies, 80 Fed. Reg. 81674 (Dec. 30, 2015). | GAO-18-341.

APPENDIX II: EXPENDITURE DATA FOR ITEMS AND SERVICES SUBJECT TO PRIOR AUTHORIZATION

Tables 4 through 7 present monthly expenditures for items and services subject to prior authorization in initial demonstration states, expansion demonstration states, and non-demonstration states from 6 months prior to each demonstration's implementation through March 2017, the most recent month for which reliable data is available.

Table 4. Monthly Power Mobility Device Expenditures from March 2012 through March 2017, by Initial Demonstration States, Expansion Demonstration States, and Non-Demonstration States

Dollars in millions

	Category	Jan	Feb	Mar	Apr	May	Jun	Jul	Aug	Sep	Oct	Nov	Dec
2012	Initial demonstration states[a]	na	na	$14.9	$14.5	$14.8	$14.2	$13.9	$14.3	$11.5	$10.3	$9.3	$8.5
	Expansion demonstration states[b]	na	na	11.6	11.6	11.7	11.2	11.0	11.2	10.4	10.2	9.6	9.3
	Non-demonstration states[c]	na	na	11.0	10.8	10.8	10.6	10.3	10.3	9.7	9.8	9.3	9.0
2013	Initial demonstration states	$7.6	$7.2	6.4	6.2	5.7	5.4	4.5	4.0	3.1	2.9	2.9	3.1
	Expansion demonstration states	8.5	8.0	7.5	6.9	6.4	6.0	5.1	4.8	3.7	3.3	3.0	3.0
	Non-demonstration states	8.3	8.0	7.4	6.9	6.4	6.1	5.5	4.9	4.0	3.6	3.4	3.4
2014	Initial demonstration states	2.6	2.5	2.5	2.6	2.8	2.8	2.8	2.8	2.9	3.1	3.0	3.0
	Expansion demonstration states	2.6	2.6	2.6	2.6	2.6	2.7	2.9	3.0	3.1	2.9	2.5	2.4
	Non-demonstration states	3.0	2.9	3.0	3.0	3.1	3.1	3.1	3.1	3.2	3.3	3.2	3.2
2015	Initial demonstration states	2.9	2.9	3.0	2.9	2.9	2.9	3.1	3.1	3.1	3.3	3.2	3.4
	Expansion demonstration states	2.3	2.3	2.4	2.3	2.4	2.4	2.5	2.5	2.6	2.6	2.6	2.9
	Non-demonstration states	3.1	3.0	3.1	3.1	3.1	3.1	3.2	3.3	3.6	3.5	3.4	3.5
2016	Initial demonstration states	2.7	2.8	2.9	2.8	2.8	2.9	2.0	1.9	2.2	2.3	2.3	2.4
	Expansion demonstration states	2.2	2.3	2.4	2.3	2.3	2.5	1.6	1.4	1.7	1.8	1.8	1.8
	Non-demonstration states	2.7	2.8	2.9	2.8	2.8	3.0	2.0	1.8	2.2	2.2	2.2	2.3
2017	Initial demonstration states	1.9	2.0	1.9	na	na	na	na	na	na	na	na	na
	Expansion demonstration states	1.6	1.6	1.7	na	na	na	na	na	na	na	na	na
	Non-demonstration states	2.0	1.8	2.0	na	na	na	na	na	na	na	na	na

Source: GAO analysis of Centers for Medicare & Medicaid Services data. | GAO-18-341.

Note: This analysis includes the 50 states and the District of Columbia.

[a]Demonstration initially implemented in September 2012 in 7 states: California, Florida, Illinois, Michigan, New York, North Carolina, and Texas.

[b]Demonstration expanded in October 2014 to 12 additional states: Arizona, Georgia, Indiana, Kentucky, Louisiana, Maryland, Missouri, New Jersey, Ohio, Pennsylvania, Tennessee, and Washington.

[c]There are 32 non-demonstration states for the demonstration.

Table 5. Monthly Repetitive Scheduled Non-Emergency Ambulance Services Expenditures from June 2014 through March 2017, by Initial Demonstration States, Expansion Demonstration States, and Non-Demonstration States

Dollars in millions

	Category	Jan	Feb	Mar	Apr	May	Jun	Jul	Aug	Sep	Oct	Nov	Dec
2014	Initial demonstration states[a]	NA	NA	NA	NA	NA	$18.7	$19.8	$18.7	$18.7	$19.4	$16.8	$11.6
	Expansion demonstration states[b]	NA	NA	NA	NA	NA	5.5	5.9	5.6	5.5	5.7	5.1	5.9
	Non-demonstration states[c]	NA	NA	NA	NA	NA	38.5	40.6	39.4	39.5	41.1	36.4	40.0
2015	Initial demonstration states	$5.6	$5.3	$6.1	$6.2	$6.3	6.3	6.4	6.1	6.1	6.3	5.8	6.2
	Expansion demonstration states	5.7	5.1	5.8	6.0	5.9	6.0	6.2	5.9	5.7	5.9	5.4	5.6
	Non-demonstration states	37.9	35.8	39.4	39.2	38.7	38.5	38.8	36.1	35.3	36.4	33.4	35.8
2016	Initial demonstration states	5.8	5.9	6.4	5.7	5.9	6.0	5.9	6.3	6.1	6.0	6.0	6.1
	Expansion demonstration states	3.4	3.3	3.6	3.3	3.3	3.4	3.3	3.3	3.1	3.1	3.1	3.2
	Non-demonstration states	33.6	33.2	34.8	33.3	33.0	32.5	32.0	34.1	32.3	32.2	31.7	32.6
2017	Initial demonstration states	5.9	5.6	6.2	NA	NA	NA	NA	NA	NA	NA	NA	NA
	Expansion demonstration states	3.0	3.1	3.3	NA	NA	NA	NA	NA	NA	NA	NA	NA
	Non-demonstration states	31.0	29.5	33.4	NA	NA	NA	NA	NA	NA	NA	NA	NA

Source: GAO analysis of Centers for Medicare & Medicaid Services data. | GAO-18-341.

Note: This analysis includes the 50 states and the District of Columbia.

[a] Demonstration initially implemented in December 2014 in 3 states: New Jersey, Pennsylvania, and South Carolina.

[b] Demonstration expanded in January 2016 to 6 additional states: Delaware, District of Columbia, Maryland, North Carolina, Virginia, and West Virginia.

[c] There are 42 non-demonstration states for the demonstration.

Table 6. Monthly Non-Emergency Hyperbaric Oxygen Therapy Expenditures from September 2014 through March 2017, by Initial Demonstration States and Non-Demonstration States

Dollars in millions

	Category	Jan	Feb	Mar	Apr	May	Jun	Jul	Aug	Sep	Oct	Nov	Dec
2014	Initial demonstration states[a]	na	na	na	na	na	na	na	na	$1.8	$1.9	$1.6	$1.6
	Non-demonstration states[b]	na	na	na	na	na	na	na	na	14.2	14.9	11.6	13.1
2015	Initial demonstration states	$1.6	$1.7	$1.7	$1.4	$1.4	$1.5	$1.5	$0.9	1.0	1.1	1.0	1.0
	Non-demonstration states	12.7	12.6	15.1	15.0	13.7	15.0	15.2	14.2	14.0	12.0	10.6	11.2
2016	Initial demonstration states	0.9	0.9	1.0	0.9	0.9	0.9	0.7	0.9	0.7	0.8	0.7	0.7
	Non-demonstration states	10.4	11.3	13.3	12.2	12.1	11.3	10.1	11.9	10.9	10.4	10.5	10.2
2017	Initial demonstration states	0.6	0.7	0.8	na	na	na	na	na	na	na	na	na
	Non-demonstration states	10.4	10.4	11.9	na	na	na	na	na	na	na	na	na

Source: GAO analysis of Centers for Medicare & Medicaid Services data. | GAO-18-341.

Note: This analysis includes the 50 states and the District of Columbia.

[a] Demonstration implemented in March 2015 in 3 states: Illinois, Michigan, and New Jersey.

[b] There are 48 non-demonstration states for the demonstration.

Table 7. Monthly Home Health Services Expenditures from February 2016 through March 2017, by Initial Demonstration States and Non-Demonstration States

Dollars in millions

	Category	Jan	Feb	Mar	Apr	May	Jun	Jul	Aug	Sep	Oct	Nov	Dec
2016	Initial demonstration states[a]	NA	$74.9	$82.8	$79.5	$78.4	$75.8	$77.1	$64.9	$62.7	$64.9	$63.8	$66.7
	Non-demonstration states[b]	NA	1,279.3	1,444.6	1,417.6	1,399.0	1,384.1	1,379.3	1,426.2	1,378.8	1,408.5	1,307.1	1,349.9
2017	Initial demonstration states	$69.0	61.5	66.9	NA	NA	NA	NA	NA	NA	NA	NA	NA
	Non-demonstration states	1,416.2	1,282.4	1,414.7	NA	NA	NA	NA	NA	NA	NA	NA	NA

Source: GAO analysis of Centers for Medicare & Medicaid Services data. | GAO-18-341.

Note: This analysis includes the 50 states and the District of Columbia.

[a]Demonstration implemented in August 2016 in 1 state: Illinois.

[b]There are 50 non-demonstration states for the demonstration.

Appendix III: Comments from the Department of Health and Human Services

Department of Health & Human Services
Office of the Secretary
Assistant Secretary for Legislation
Washington DC 20201
Mar 30, 2018

Kathleen King
Director, Health Care
U.S. Government Accountability Office
441 G Street NW
Washington, DC 20548

Dear Ms. King:

Attached are comments on the U.S. Government Accountability Office's (GAO) report entitled, *"Medicare: CMS Should Take Actions to Continue Prior Authorization Efforts to Reduce Spending"* (GAO-18-341).

The Department appreciates the opportunity to review this report to publication.

Sincerely,
Matthew D. Bassett
Assistant Secretary for Legislation

General Comments from the Department of Health and Human Services on the Government Accountability Office's Draft Report Entitled- Medicare: CMS Should Take Actions to Continue Prior Authorization Efforts to Reduce Spending (GAO-18-341)

The U.S. Department of Health and Human Services (HHS) appreciates the opportunity from the Government Accountability Office (GAO) to review and comment on this draft report. HHS is committed to providing Medicare beneficiaries with access to high quality health care while protecting taxpayer dollars.

As part of HHS's program integrity strategy, HHS implemented several prior authorization programs, including one permanent program and three demonstrations/models. Prior authorization is a process through which a request for provisional affirmation of coverage is submitted for review before an item or service is furnished to a beneficiary and before a claim is submitted for payment. Prior authorization helps to make sure that applicable coverage, payment, and coding rules are met before items and services are furnished. HHS also implemented one pre-claim review program. Pre-claim review is a process through which a request for provisional affirmation of coverage is submitted for review before a final claim is submitted for payment. Pre-claim review helps make sure that applicable coverage, payment, and coding rules are met before the final claim is submitted.

Two of the Medicare prior authorization programs (repetitive, scheduled non-emergent ambulance transport and non-emergent hyperbaric oxygen therapy) were models developed to reduce expenditures, while maintaining or improving quality of care. One of the Medicare prior authorization programs (power mobility devices) and the Medicare pre-claim review program (home health services) were demonstrations that helped develop or demonstrate improved methods for the investigation and prosecution of fraud in the provision of care or services. Pursuant to section 1834(a)(1 5) of the Social Security Act, HHS also implemented a permanent Durable Medical Equipment, Prosthetics, Orthotics, and

Supplies (DMEPOS) prior authorization program for certain DMEPOS items that are frequently subject to unnecessary utilization.

HHS has been closely monitoring the impact of the prior authorization and pre-claim review programs on beneficiaries, suppliers, providers, and Medicare expenditures to evaluate the results of each program and help inform next steps. HHS appreciates the GAO's review in this area and will consider findings from this report as we continue to evaluate the use of prior authorization and pre-claim review in Medicare.

Recommendation 1

The Administrator of the Centers for Medicare & Medicaid Services (CMS) should subject accessories essential to the group 3 power wheelchairs in the permanent DMEPOS program to prior authorization.

HHS Response

HHS continues to evaluate ways to improve the program and will take the GAO's recommendation into consideration when developing plans in this area.

Recommendation 2

The Administrator of CMS should take steps, based on results from evaluations, to continue prior authorization. These steps could include:

- resuming the paused home health services demonstration;
- extending current demonstrations; or.
- identifying new opportunities for expanding prior authorization to additional items and services with high unnecessary utilization and high improper payment rates.

HHS Response

HHS will continue to evaluate the prior authorization programs and will take the GAO's findings and recommendations into account when determining appropriate next steps.

In addition, HHS only has statutory authority to permanently require prior authorization for specified Medicare Fee-For-Service (FFS) items and services. The Fiscal Year 2019 President's Budget for HHS included a legislative proposal to extend that authority to all Medicare FFS items and services, specifically those items that are at high risk for fraud, waste, and abuse. By allowing prior authorization on additional items and services, as appropriate, HHS can ensure in advance that, in those circumstances, the correct payment goes to the right provider for the appropriate service, and avoid future audits on those payments.

APPENDIX IV: GAO CONTACT AND STAFF ACKNOWLEDGMENTS

GAO Contact

A. Nicole Clowers, (202) 512-7114
or clowersa@gao.gov

Kathleen M. King, (202) 512-7114
or kingk@gao.gov

Staff Acknowledgments

In addition to the contact named above, Martin T. Gahart (Assistant Director), Lori Achman (Assistant Director), Peter Mangano (Analyst-in-Charge), Sylvia Diaz Jones, and Mandy Pusey made key contributions to this report. Also contributing were Sam Amrhein, Muriel Brown, Eric Wedum, and Jennifer Whitworth.

APPENDIX V: ACCESSIBLE DATA

Agency Comment Letter

Text of Appendix III: Comments from the Department of Health and Human Services

Kathleen King Director, Health Care

U.S. Government Accountability Office

Dear Ms. King:

Assistant Secretary for Legislation Washington, DC 20201

Attached are comments on the U.S. Government Accountability Office's (GAO) report entitled, "Medicare: CMS Should Take Actions to Continue Prior Authorization Efforts to Reduce Spending" (GAO-18-341).

The Department appreciates the opportunity to review this report prior to publication.

Sincerely,
Matthew D. Bassett
Assistant Secretary for Legislation

The U.S. Department of Health and Human Services (HHS) appreciates the opportunity from the Government Accountability Office (GAO) to review and comment on this draft report. HHS is committed to providing Medicare beneficiaries with access to high quality health care while protecting taxpayer dollars.

As part of HHS's program integrity strategy, HHS implemented several prior authorization programs, including one permanent program and three demonstrations/models. Prior authorization is a process through which a request for provisional affirmation of coverage is submitted for review before an item or service is furnished to a beneficiary and before a claim is submitted for payment. Prior authorization helps to make sure that applicable coverage, payment, and coding rules are met before items and services are furnished. HHS also implemented one pre-claim review program. Pre-claim review is a process through which a request for provisional affirmation of coverage is submitted for review before a final claim is submitted for payment. Pre-claim review helps make sure that applicable coverage, payment, and coding rules are met before the final claim is submitted.

Two of the Medicare prior authorization programs (repetitive, scheduled non-emergent ambulance transport and non-emergent hyperbaric oxygen therapy) were models developed to reduce expenditures, while maintaining or improving quality of care. One of the Medicare prior authorization programs (power mobility devices) and the Medicare pre-claim review program (home health services) were demonstrations that helped develop or demonstrate improved methods for the investigation and prosecution of fraud in the provision of care or services.

Pursuant to section 1834(a)(l 5) of the Social Security Act, HHS also implemented a permanent Durable Medical Equipment, Prosthetics, Orthotics, and Supplies (DMEPOS) prior authorization program for certain DMEPOS items that are frequently subject to unnecessary utilization.

HHS has been closely monitoring the impact of the prior authorization and pre-claim review programs on beneficiaries, suppliers, providers, and Medicare expenditures to evaluate the results of each program and help inform next steps. HHS appreciates the GAO's review in this area and will consider findings from this report as we continue to evaluate the use of prior authorization and pre-claim review in Medicare.

Recommendation 1

The Administrator of the Centers for Medicare & Medicaid Services (CMS) should subject accessories essential to the group 3 power wheelchairs in the permanent DMEPOS program to prior authorization.

HHS Response

HHS continues to evaluate ways to improve the program and will take the GAO's recommendation into consideration when developing plans in this area.

Recommendation 2

The Administrator of CMS should take steps, based on results from evaluations, to continue prior authorization. These steps could include:

- resuming the paused home health services demonstration;
- extending current demonstrations; or.
- identifying new opportunities for expanding prior authorization to additional items and services with high unnecessary utilization and high improper payment rates.

HHS Response

HHS will continue to evaluate the prior authorization programs and will take the GAO's findings and recommendations into account when determining appropriate next steps.

In addition, HHS only has statutory authority to permanently require prior authorization for specified Medicare Fee-For-Service (FFS) items and services. The Fiscal Year 2019 President's Budget for HHS included a legislative proposal to extend that authority to all Medicare FFS items and services, specifically those items that are at high risk for fraud, waste, and abuse. By allowing prior authorization on additional items and services, as appropriate, HHS can ensure in advance that, in those circumstances, the correct payment goes to the right provider for the appropriate service, and avoid future audits on those payments.

In: Medicare: Financing, Insolvency and Fraud ISBN: 978-1-53614-811-4
Editor: Bradford Rodgers   © 2019 Nova Science Publishers, Inc.

Chapter 5

MEDICARE: CMS FRAUD PREVENTION SYSTEM USES CLAIMS ANALYSIS TO ADDRESS FRAUD[*]

United States Government Accountability Office

WHY GAO DID THIS STUDY

CMS analyzes Medicare fee-for-service claims data to further its program integrity activities. In 2011, CMS implemented a data analytic system called FPS to develop leads for fraud investigations conducted by CMS program integrity contractors and to deny improper payments. In developing leads, FPS is intended to help CMS avoid improper payment costs by enabling quicker investigations and more timely corrective actions. Additionally, in 2012, CMS helped establish the HFPP to collaborate with other health care payers to address health care fraud. One

---

[*] This is an edited, reformatted and augmented version of United States Government Accountability Office; Report to Congressional Requesters; Accessible Version, Publication No. GAO-17-710, dated August 2017.

of the key activities of the HFPP is to analyze claims data that are pooled from multiple payers, including private payers and Medicare.

GAO was asked to review CMS's use of FPS and the activities of the HFPP. This report examines 1) CMS's use of FPS to identify and investigate providers suspected of potential fraud, 2) the types of payments that have been denied by FPS, and 3) HFPP efforts to further CMS's and payers' ability to address health care fraud. GAO reviewed CMS documents, including reports to Congress on FPS, contractor statements of work, and information technology system user guides, and obtained fiscal year 2015 and 2016 data on FPS fraud investigations and claim denials. GAO also interviewed CMS officials and CMS program integrity contractors regarding how they use FPS, and a non-generalizable selection of HFPP participants regarding information and data sharing practices, and anti-fraud collaboration efforts.

WHAT GAO FOUND

Investigations initiated or supported by the Centers for Medicare & Medicaid Services' (CMS) Fraud Prevention System (FPS)—a data analytic system—led to corrective actions against providers and generated savings. For example, in fiscal year 2016, CMS reported that 90 providers had their payments suspended because of investigations initiated or supported by FPS, which resulted in an estimated $6.7 million in savings. In fiscal year 2016, 22 percent of Medicare fraud investigations conducted by CMS program integrity contractors were based on leads generated by FPS analysis of Medicare claims data. Officials representing Medicare's program integrity contractors told GAO that FPS helps speed up certain investigation processes, such as identifying and triaging suspect providers for investigation. However, the officials said that once an investigation is initiated, FPS has generally not sped up the process for investigating and gathering evidence against suspect providers. CMS has not tracked data to assess the extent to which FPS has affected the timeliness of contractor investigation processes. However, CMS is implementing a new information technology system that tracks such data, and officials said that they plan to use the data to assess FPS's effect on timeliness.

FPS denies individual claims for payment that violate Medicare rules or policies through prepayment edits—automated controls that compare claims against Medicare requirements in order to approve or deny claims. FPS prepayment edits specifically target payments associated with potential fraud. For example, an FPS edit denies physician claims that improperly increase payments by misidentifying the place that the service was rendered, which helped address a payment vulnerability associated with millions in overpayments. FPS edits do not analyze individual claims to automatically deny them based on risk alone or the likelihood that they are fraudulent without further investigation. As of May 2017, CMS had implemented 24 edits in FPS. CMS reported that FPS edits denied nearly 324,000 claims and saved more than $20.4 million in fiscal year 2016.

The Healthcare Fraud Prevention Partnership (HFPP) is a public-private partnership that began in 2012 with the aim of facilitating collaboration among health care payers to address health care fraud. The HFPP had 79 participants as of June 2017. Participants, including CMS officials, stated that sharing data and information within HFPP has been useful to their efforts to address health care fraud. HFPP conducts studies that pool and analyze multiple payers' claims data to identify providers with patterns of suspect billing across payers. Participants reported that HFPP's studies helped them to identify and take action against potentially fraudulent providers and payment vulnerabilities of which they might not otherwise have been aware. For example, one study identified providers who were cumulatively billing multiple payers for more services than could reasonably be rendered in a single day. Participants also stated that HFPP has fostered both formal and informal information sharing among payers.

The Department of Health and Human Services provided technical comments on a draft of this report, which GAO incorporated as appropriate.

ABBREVIATIONS

CMS	Centers for Medicare & Medicaid Services
CPI	Center for Program Integrity
FPS	Fraud Prevention System
HFPP	Healthcare Fraud Prevention Partnership
HHS	Department of Health and Human Services
HHS OIG	Department of Health and Human Services Office of Inspector General
IT	information technology
MAC	Medicare Administrative Contractor
TTP	trusted third party
UPIC	Unified Program Integrity Contractor
ZPIC	Zone Program Integrity Contractor

441 G St. N.W.
Washington, DC 20548
August 30, 2017
Congressional Requesters

In fiscal year 2016, Medicare provided health insurance for approximately 57 million elderly and disabled beneficiaries at a cost of approximately $699 billion.[1] Since 1990, we have designated Medicare a high-risk program because of its size, complexity, and susceptibility to mismanagement and improper payments.[2] Some improper Medicare

---

[1] Medicare is the federally financed health insurance program for persons aged 65 and over, certain individuals with disabilities, and individuals with end-stage renal disease. Medicare Part A covers inpatient hospital services, skilled nursing facility services, some home health services, and hospice services. Medicare Part B covers physician and hospital outpatient services, and durable medical equipment, prosthetics, orthotics, and supplies, among other things. Together, Parts A and B are known as traditional Medicare or Medicare fee-for-service.

[2] See GAO, *High-Risk Series: Progress on Many High-Risk Areas, While Substantial Efforts Needed on Others*, GAO-17-317 (Washington, D.C.: Feb. 15, 2017).

payments are due to fraud, which involves willful misrepresentation.[3] Although the deceptive nature of fraud makes its extent in the Medicare program difficult to measure in a reliable way, there have been convictions for multimillion dollar schemes defrauding the program.

The Centers for Medicare & Medicaid Services (CMS)—the agency within the Department of Health and Human Services (HHS) that administers the Medicare program—is responsible for conducting program integrity activities intended to reduce fraud, waste, and abuse. CMS uses analyses of claims submitted for payment by health care providers as part of its program integrity activities. In 2011, CMS implemented a data analytic system—the Fraud Prevention System (FPS)—that analyzes Medicare fee-for-service claims to identify health care providers with suspect billing patterns for further investigation and to prevent improper payments. Additionally, in 2012, HHS helped establish a public-private partnership—the Healthcare Fraud Prevention Partnership (HFPP)—with other health care payers, agencies, and organizations to address healthcare fraud. One of the key activities of HFPP is analyzing claims data pooled from multiple payers, including Medicare, to identify and disseminate information within the partnership on providers with suspect billing patterns.

You asked us to review CMS's use of FPS and the activities of HFPP. This report examines

1) CMS's use of FPS to identify and investigate providers suspected of potential fraud;

---

[3] The Medicare fee-for-service program generally makes payments directly to health care providers, such as hospitals and physicians. An improper payment is any payment that should not have been made or that was made in an incorrect amount (including overpayments and underpayments) under statutory, contractual, administrative, or other legally applicable requirements. This includes any payment to an ineligible recipient, any payment for an ineligible good or service, any duplicate payment, any payment for a good or service not received (except for such payments where authorized by law), and any payment that does not account for credit for applicable discounts. Improper payments may be a result of fraud, waste, or abuse. Fraud involves an intentional act or representation to deceive with the knowledge that the actions or representation could result in gain. Whether an act is in fact fraud is a determination that is made through the judicial or other adjudicative system. Waste includes overusing services, such as excessive diagnostic testing. Abuse involves actions inconsistent with acceptable business or medical practices.

2) the types of payments that have been denied by FPS; and
3) HFPP's efforts to further CMS's and payers' ability to address health care fraud.

To examine CMS's use of FPS to identify and investigate suspect providers, we reviewed CMS documents, including CMS reports to Congress on FPS's implementation, statements of work for program integrity contractors, and FPS and other CMS information technology (IT) system user guides. We interviewed CMS officials and officials from all seven Zone Program Integrity Contractors (ZPIC)—the contractors responsible for identifying and investigating potential Medicare fraud, waste, and abuse—regarding how FPS is used to identify and investigate potential fraud.[4] CMS is currently in the process of transitioning Medicare program integrity contracts from ZPICs to new contract entities, Unified Program Integrity Contractors (UPIC), and we interviewed officials from the two UPICs in operation as of May 2017.[5] We also obtained and analyzed fiscal year 2015 and 2016 data from CMS on the sources of ZPIC investigations and the corrective actions and savings associated with ZPIC investigations. To assess the reliability of the data, we reviewed relevant agency documents, interviewed CMS officials, compared the data to published data, and reviewed the data for any outliers and obvious errors. We found the data sufficiently reliable for the purposes of our study.

To examine the types of payments that have been denied by FPS, we obtained information from CMS on the prepayment edits—automated controls that compare claim information to Medicare coverage and payment policies in order to approve or deny claims—that have been

---

[4] CMS began implementing ZPICs in 2008 to replace legacy program integrity contractors, Program Safeguard Contractors. Program Safeguard Contractors continued to operate in one ZPIC jurisdiction— Zone 6—because of protest-related delays with the Zone 6 ZPIC contract. We interviewed officials representing the Program Safeguard Contractors that operated in Zone 6. For the sake of simplicity, references to ZPICs in this report are inclusive of the Zone 6 Program Safeguard Contractors.

[5] UPICs combine responsibility for conducting program integrity activities for both the Medicare and Medicaid programs. CMS plans to award all UPIC contracts by the end of calendar year 2017.

implemented in FPS.[6] We interviewed CMS officials about how FPS's edits identify and deny payments. We also interviewed officials representing Medicare Administrative Contractors (MAC)—the contractors that process and pay Medicare fee-for-service claims and, along with CMS, are responsible for implementing prepayment edits—regarding differences between edits in FPS and those in Medicare's claims processing systems. In addition, we obtained data from CMS on the number of claims denied by FPS edits and the associated savings for fiscal years 2015 and 2016. To assess the reliability of the data, we interviewed CMS officials, compared the data to published data, and reviewed the data for any outliers and obvious errors. We found the data sufficiently reliable for the purposes of our study.

To examine HFPP's efforts to further CMS's and payers' ability to address health care fraud, we reviewed CMS and HFPP documents, including HFPP study summaries and findings. We interviewed officials from CMS and the contractors that have administered HFPP about HFPP information and data sharing practices. We also interviewed a non-generalizable selection of HFPP participants that reflect HFPP's membership. We interviewed officials representing 3 private payers, 5 state agencies, and 4 associations regarding HFPP's anti-fraud collaboration efforts. We selected private payers that offer Medicare Advantage plans, state agencies that use data analytic systems or have shared data for HFPP studies, and healthcare and healthcare fraud specific associations.

We conducted this performance audit from April 2016 to August 2017 in accordance with generally accepted government auditing standards. Those standards require that we plan and perform the audit to obtain sufficient, appropriate evidence to provide a reasonable basis for our findings and conclusions based on our audit objectives. We believe that the evidence obtained provides a reasonable basis for our findings and conclusions based on our audit objectives.

---

[6] References to FPS claim denials refer to both claims that are rejected or denied by the system. Claims that are rejected can be corrected and resubmitted, while claims that are denied cannot be resubmitted.

BACKGROUND

Fraud Prevention System

To advance CMS's efforts to prevent fraud, waste, and abuse in the Medicare fee-for service program, the Small Business Jobs Act of 2010 appropriated $100 million for CMS to implement a data analytic system.[7] The law required CMS to implement a system that could analyze claims prior to payment to identify suspect claims and provider billing patterns and prevent payment of improper and potentially fraudulent claims, among other things. In April 2011, CMS awarded almost $77 million to a contractor to implement, operate, and maintain FPS and design analytic models for the system. CMS awarded about $13 million to a second contractor in July 2011 to develop additional analytic models for FPS. As the original FPS contract was set to end, CMS awarded a nearly $92 million contract in April 2016 for a new, upgraded FPS system—FPS 2.0. FPS 2.0 was fully implemented in March 2017.

CMS's Center for Program Integrity (CPI)—which oversees the agency's Medicare program integrity efforts—employs FPS as a key component of its strategy to move beyond the "pay and chase" approach of recovering improper and potentially fraudulent payments to focusing on prevention. FPS screens fee-for-service claims prior to payment in order to help identify and prevent improper and potentially fraudulent payments by performing two primary functions:

- *Develop leads for fraud investigations.* FPS compares provider billing patterns and other data against models of potentially

---

[7] A portion of the appropriated funds was required to be used for an independent evaluation of the program. Pub. L. No. 111-240, § 4241(h), 124 Stat. 2504, 2603 (2010) (codified at 42 U.S.C. § 1320a-7m(h)). Data analytic systems are IT systems that use a variety of techniques to analyze and interpret data to facilitate decision making, and can be used to identify patterns or trends. We have previously reported on the importance of agencies using data analysis to manage fraud risks. See GAO, *A Framework for Managing Fraud Risks in Federal Programs*, GAO-15-593SP (Washington, D.C.: July 2015) and GAO, *Highlights of a Forum: Data Analytics to Address Fraud and Improper Payments*, GAO-17-339SP (Washington, D.C.: Mar. 31, 2017).

fraudulent behavior to identify providers with suspect billing patterns. For example, an FPS model identifies providers that bill for a disproportionate number of services in a single day relative to other providers. FPS simultaneously risk-scores providers identified by the models to prioritize them for potential investigation. In developing these leads, FPS is intended to help CMS prevent potentially fraudulent payments by furthering the agency's ability to more quickly identify and investigate suspect providers, and take more timely corrective actions.

- *Execute automated prepayment edits.* FPS edits deny certain improper payments, and some edits compare information from multiple claims to do so. For example, FPS may deny physician outpatient claims based on information from an inpatient claim associated with the same episode of care.

CMS submitted three annual reports on FPS's implementation to Congress in response to requirements established by the Small Business Jobs Act of 2010. In these reports, CMS provided information on the corrective actions taken and savings achieved from FPS.[8] In its most recent report, CMS reported that FPS had cumulatively helped prevent or identify nearly $1.5 billion in improper and potentially fraudulent payments from its implementation through the end of calendar year 2015.[9]

---

[8] The act further required HHS Office of Inspector General (HHS OIG) to certify the reported savings from FPS, and HHS OIG issued companion reports on CMS's reported savings for the first three years of FPS. Although not required by the act to report on FPS after the first three years, CMS publicly issued a fourth year report. See https://w ww.cms.gov/About-CMS/Components/CPI/Downloads/Fraud-Prevention-SystemReturn-on-Investment-Fourth-Implementation-Year-2015.pdf.

[9] The $1.5 billion figure above includes both payments directly prevented by FPS, such as prepayment edit claim denials, and identified savings associated with actions taken against providers suspected of fraud, such as the amount of overpayments referred for collection. The actual savings achieved is lower because of a number of factors. For example, not all referred overpayments can be recovered. CMS applies adjustment factors to the identified savings to estimate actual savings from FPS. For instance, while CMS reported $454 million in prevented and identified savings from FPS in calendar year 2014, CMS estimated actual savings of $133 million. For more information on the adjustment factors used by CMS, see CMS, *Report to Congress Fraud Prevention System Second Implementation Year*, June 2014.

Medicare Program Integrity

CMS uses contractors to support the agency's program integrity activities, including program integrity contractors to identify and investigate providers engaged in potential Medicare fee-for-service fraud. CMS is currently in the process of transitioning Medicare program integrity contracts from ZPICs to new contract entities, UPICs. ZPICs operated in seven geographical jurisdictions across the country. UPICs will operate in five jurisdictions and combine Medicare and Medicaid program integrity efforts under a single contracting entity (Figure 1 depicts the geographic jurisdictions of ZPIC and UPIC zones). As of May 2017, two of the five UPICs—the Midwestern and Northeastern—were operational.

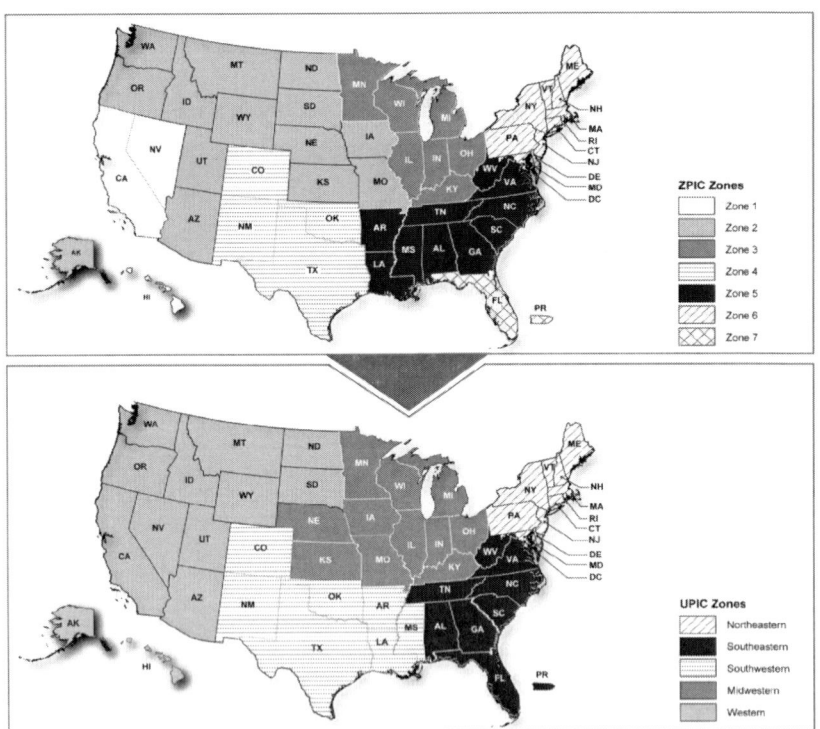

Source: CMS; Map Resources (map). | GAO-17-710.

Figure 1. Zone Program Integrity Contractor (ZPIC) and Unified Program Integrity Contractor (UPIC) Jurisdictions.

The program integrity contractors identify leads for provider investigations from three categories of sources:

- *Referrals.* A number of entities, including CMS, law enforcement agencies, and the MACs, refer leads about suspect providers to the program integrity contractors. The program integrity contractors also receive leads based on beneficiary and provider complaints and allegations.
- *Program integrity contractor data analysis.* Program integrity contractors use post-payment claims to conduct their own data analyses to identify providers with suspect billing patterns.
- *FPS.* FPS identifies providers with suspect billing patterns and prioritizes leads based on provider risk-scores.

The program integrity contractors generally have a triage process to review leads and determine whether the leads are indicative of potential fraud (see fig. 2 for information on program integrity contractor investigation processes). Leads that are determined to be suspect become formal investigations, and the program integrity contractors perform a range of investigative activities to gather evidence and determine if providers are engaged in potential fraud. These activities include conducting beneficiary and provider interviews, site visits of provider facilities, and manual reviews of provider claims.

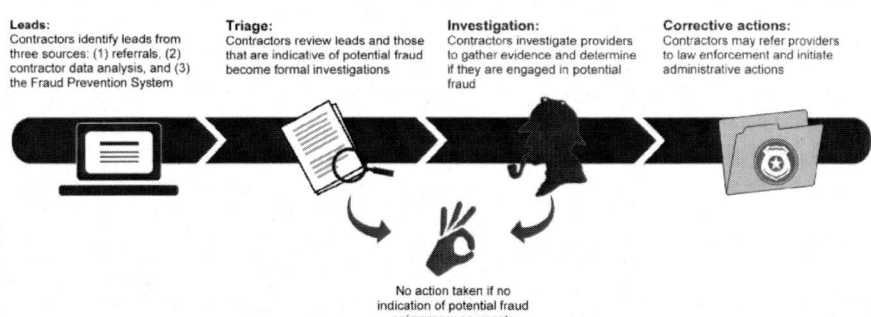

Source: GAO analysis of CMS information. | GAO-17-710.

Figure 2. Program Integrity Contractor Investigation Processes.

Table 1. Administrative Actions against Medicare Providers That May Result from Program Integrity Investigations

Action	Definition
Prepayment review	Provider-specific prepayment edits that suspend payments pending manual claim review.
Provider-specific auto-denial edits	Provider-specific prepayment edits that automatically deny payments to the provider.
Payment suspension	Temporary suspension of provider payments pending investigation of potential fraud.
Overpayment determination	Referral for collection of provider payments received in excess of amounts due and payable.
Revocation	Termination of provider's billing privileges.

Source: GAO analysis of CMS information. | GAO-17-710.

Based on their investigations, the program integrity contractors may take corrective actions by referring providers engaged in potential fraud to law enforcement and initiating administrative actions. Specifically, if the program integrity contractors uncover evidence of potential fraud, they refer the investigation to the Department of Health and Human Services Office of Inspector General (HHS OIG) for further examination, which may lead to possible criminal or civil prosecution by the Department of Justice. The program integrity contractors may also recommend a range of administrative actions to CMS for approval and implementation. Such actions include revocation of providers' billing privileges and payment suspensions (Table 1 describes the administrative actions the program integrity contractors may recommend against providers).

CMS's Prepayment Edits Process

CMS's claims processing systems apply prepayment edits to all Medicare fee-for-service claims in an effort to pay claims properly. Most of the prepayment edits are automated, meaning that if a claim does not meet the criteria of the edit, it is automatically denied. Other prepayment edits flag claims for manual review, in which trained clinicians and coders examine claims and associated medical records to ensure that the claims meet Medicare rules and requirements. Many improper and potentially fraudulent claims can be identified only by manually reviewing associated medical records and beneficiary claim histories, and exercising clinical judgment to determine whether services were reasonable and necessary. Whereas automated edits are applied to all claims, manual edits are applied to very few—less than 1 percent of claims undergo manual review.

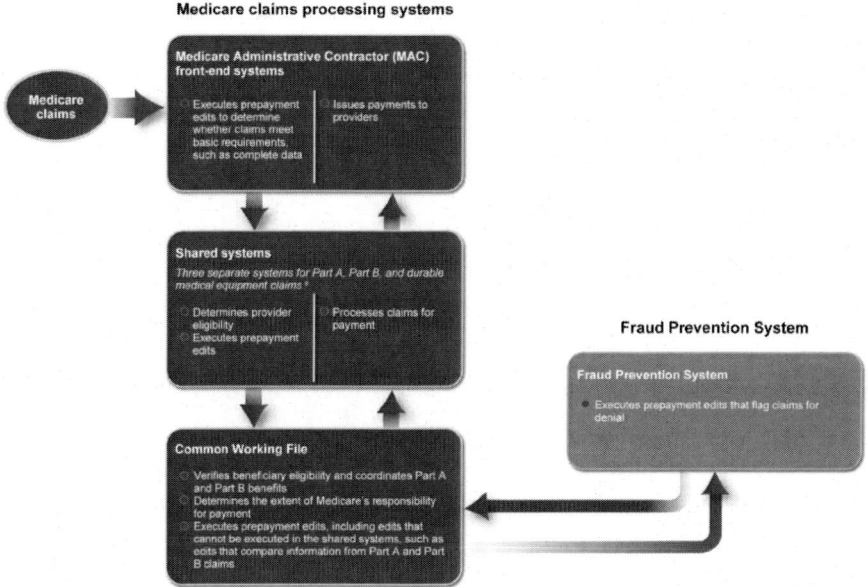

Source: GAO analysis of CMS information. | GAO-17-710.

[a]The shared systems are the Fiscal Intermediary Shared System, Multi-Carrier System, and the ViPS Medicare System. The Fiscal Intermediary Shared System processes Part A claims and certain Part B claims related to medical care provided by institutional providers, such as hospital inpatient and outpatient departments. The Multi-Carrier System processes all other Part B claims, such as physician claims. The ViPS Medicare System processes claims for durable medical equipment.

Figure 3. Medicare Claims Processing.

CMS contracts with the MACs to process and pay Medicare fee-for-service claims and implement prepayment edits in the Medicare claims processing systems.[10] The claims processing systems consist of three systems—the MAC front-end systems, shared systems, and Common Working File—that carry out a variety of functions and execute prepayment edits (see Figure 3). When implementing FPS, CMS integrated FPS with the claims processing systems and claims are screened by FPS prior to payment. Unlike the claims processing systems, CPI maintains FPS.

Healthcare Fraud Prevention Partnership

HFPP is a voluntary public-private partnership established by HHS and the Department of Justice to facilitate collaboration in addressing healthcare fraud. The membership includes Medicare- and Medicaid-related federal agencies and several state agencies, other federal agencies with responsibility for federal health care programs such as the Department of Defense and Department of Veterans Affairs, law enforcement agencies, private payers, and antifraud and other healthcare organizations. HFPP was established, in part, to help payers identify schemes and providers engaged in potential fraud that individual payers may not be able to identify alone. HFPP began in 2012 with 20 members and, as of June 2017, had grown to 79 members.[11] As of the end of calendar year 2016, CMS had cumulatively spent $30.3 million on HFPP.

---

[10] CMS is generally required to pay Medicare claims between 14 and 30 days from the date of receipt.

[11] In November 2016, HFPP had 70 members and CMS reported that payer participants covered approximately 65 percent of covered U.S. individuals.

CMS PROGRAM INTEGRITY CONTRACTORS REPORTED THAT FPS SPEEDS UP CERTAIN INVESTIGATION PROCESSES AND HAS CONTRIBUTED TO PROGRAM SAVINGS

CMS Program Integrity Contractors Reported That FPS Speeds Up Certain Investigation Processes, and CMS Is Taking Steps to Track Data on Timeliness

ZPIC officials stated that FPS helps them identify suspect providers quickly. Because FPS analyzes claims prior to payment, providers with suspect billing patterns can be identified quickly relative to other sources of leads. In particular, several ZPIC officials stated that the leads they develop from their data analyses of post-payment claims are not as timely. Officials from two ZPICs estimated that the post-payment claims they use for their analyses may have been for services rendered 1 to 2 months prior, while the claims analyzed by FPS may have been for services recently rendered.

ZPIC officials also said the information associated with FPS leads allows them to examine and triage those leads quickly to determine whether to initiate investigations. FPS leads provide specific information about the type of potential fraud identified, along with claims data and other supporting information. ZPIC officials further stated that they use information from FPS when triaging leads from other sources. In contrast to FPS leads, several ZPIC officials noted that reviewing and triaging leads based on referrals often necessitates additional time and resources. In particular, allegations associated with some referrals can be vague, which makes it difficult for ZPICs to identify the relevant provider claims data and other information needed to assess the validity of the allegations.

However, once an investigation is initiated, officials stated that FPS has generally not sped up the process for investigating providers. Several ZPIC officials noted that investigations based on FPS leads are similar to those from other sources in that they require further investigation, such as manual claim reviews or site visits of provider facilities, to substantiate the leads and gather evidence of potential fraud. However, while ZPIC officials said that FPS does not speed up investigations, officials from several ZPICs noted that FPS can help improve the quality of beneficiary interviews. Since FPS leads are based on prepayment claims data, ZPICs can conduct beneficiary interviews shortly after the services have been rendered, when beneficiaries may be better able to recall details about their care.

CMS has not tracked data to assess FPS's effect on the timeliness of investigation processes.[12] CMS has lacked such timeliness data because of limitations with its IT system for managing and overseeing ZPICs. However, as of May 2017, CMS was in the process of implementing a new IT system that could be used to assess FPS's effect on the timeliness of program integrity contractor investigation processes. In transitioning to UPICs, CMS is implementing a new contractor workload management system that will capture data on the timeliness of UPIC investigation processes.[13] For example, the system will be able to capture information on the amount of time it takes a UPIC to evaluate a lead or conduct an investigation. CMS officials said that the agency plans to use the information tracked by the system to monitor program performance, including assessing FPS's effect on UPIC investigation processes and the timeliness of corrective actions. The officials also stated that they may not be able to conduct such an assessment for several years as CMS is still in the process of transitioning to UPICs and implementing the new IT system. Further, the officials said that they subsequently would want to collect several years' worth of such data to ensure a reliable assessment.

---

[12] We previously reported on the importance of tracking the timeliness of program integrity contractor investigation processes, since CMS can save money by taking administrative actions against providers suspected of fraud more quickly. See GAO, *Medicare Program Integrity: Contractors Reported Generating Savings, but CMS Could Improve Its Oversight*, GAO-14-111 (Washington, D.C.: Oct. 25, 2013).

[13] CMS is replacing the Analysis, Reporting, and Tracking system used by ZPICs with the Unified Case Management system for UPICs.

FPS Accounted for About 20 Percent of Investigations in 2015 and 2016 and Contributed to Program Savings

In fiscal years 2015 and 2016, about 20 percent of ZPIC investigations were initiated based on FPS leads, according to our analysis (see Table 2). In both years, nearly half of ZPIC investigations were based on referrals.

The proportion of investigations based on FPS leads is poised to increase as CMS changes program integrity contractor requirements for using FPS with the transition from ZPICs to UPICs. CMS has required the ZPICs to review all FPS leads that met high-risk thresholds. CMS is instead requiring that the UPICs derive 45 percent of new investigations from FPS. ZPIC officials stated that the new UPIC requirement should allow UPICs flexibility to focus their reviews on the FPS leads that are most applicable to their geographic region. For example, a UPIC with high levels of home health agency fraud within its jurisdiction can focus its reviews of FPS leads on those providers.[14]

Table 2. Sources of Zone Program Integrity Contractor (ZPIC) Investigations, Fiscal Years (FY) 2015 and 2016

Source of investigations	FY 2015		FY 2016	
	Number of new investigations	Percentage of workload	Number of new investigations	Percentage of workload
Referrals	1513	53	1395	47
ZPIC data analysis	722	25	937	31
FPS	604	21	654	22

Source: GAO analysis of CMS data. | GAO-17-710.
Note: Percentages may not sum to 100 due to rounding.

---

[14] We previously found CMS's requirement that ZPICs review all FPS leads that met high-risk thresholds created challenges for ZPICs because FPS sometimes prioritized leads that targeted fraud schemes that were not prevalent in specific ZPIC zones. See GAO, *Medicare Fraud Prevention: CMS Has Implemented a Predictive Analytics System, but Needs to Define Measures to Determine Its Effectiveness*, GAO-13-104 (Washington, D.C.: Oct. 15, 2012).

Table 3. CMS Reported Program Integrity Contractor Corrective Actions and Associated Savings from FPS, Fiscal Years (FY) 2015 and 2016

Action		FY 2015			FY 2016		
	Total actions	Actions associated with FPS[a]	Percentage associated with FPS	Total actions	Actions associated with FPS[a]	Percentage associated with FPS
Number of providers subject to prepayment review	546	311	57%	686	446	65%
Estimated savings[b] (dollars in millions)	$59.8	$15.0	25%	$54.0	$17.3	32%
Number of providers subject to auto-denial edits[c]	—	236	—	—	238	—
Estimated savings[b] (dollars in millions)	$63.4	$1.5	2%	$54.5	$1.7	3%
Number of overpayment determinations referred for collection	876	443	51%	1112	526	47%
Amount referred for collection (dollars in millions)	$935.7	$291.7	31%	$1221.2	$358.8	29%
Estimated savings[d] (dollars in millions)	$175.5	$40.0	23%	$178.7	$52.7	29%
Number of providers subject to payment suspension during the fiscal year	377	55	15%	393	90	23%
Estimated savings[e] (dollars in millions)	$49.7	$12.9	26%	$46.7	$6.7	14%
Number of providers revoked	441	101	23%	303	45	15%
Number of providers referred to law enforcement[f]	—	53	—	—	41	—

Source: GAO analysis of Centers for Medicare & Medicaid Services (CMS) data. | GAO-17-710.

Notes: CMS applies adjustment factors to identified savings amounts to estimate actual savings. For more information on the adjustment factors used by CMS, see CMS, Report to Congress Fraud Prevention System Second Implementation Year, June 2014.

[a]Includes both actions from investigations initiated by the Fraud Prevention System (FPS) and existing investigations that were supported or corroborated by FPS.

[b]The savings amounts are estimates of what CMS would have paid had the claims been processed, and are further adjusted based on the historic rate at which claim denials are overturned on appeal.

[c]For the total actions, CMS tracked the number of auto-denial edits implemented. For actions associated with FPS, CMS tracked the number of providers subject to auto-denial edits. These data are not directly comparable.

[d]The savings amounts are estimates based on historic overpayment collection rates, with the exception of the total amount collected in FY 2016. Starting in FY 2016, CMS began tracking total overpayment savings based on actual amounts collected.

Medicare 135

ᵉThe savings amounts are estimates based on the historic rate at which payments held in suspension because of program integrity contractor actions are later recouped.

ᶠFor total actions, CMS tracked the number of investigations referred to law enforcement. For actions associated with FPS, CMS tracked the number of providers referred to law enforcement. These data are not directly comparable.

Investigations initiated by FPS and existing investigations that were supported by FPS have led to corrective actions against providers engaged in potential fraud and program savings, based on CMS reported data. For example, in fiscal year 2015, nearly 60 percent of providers subject to prepayment review and 25 percent of estimated savings from prepayment reviews were associated with FPS (see Table 3). In fiscal year 2016, nearly 25 percent of provider payment suspensions and about 15 percent of estimated savings from payment suspensions were associated with FPS.

In addition to tracking the corrective actions and savings associated with FPS, CMS also measures the extent to which investigations initiated from FPS leads result in actions against providers engaged in potential fraud.[15] CMS reported that, in fiscal year 2015, 44 percent of FPS-initiated investigations resulted in administrative actions, which met the agency's fiscal year goal of 42 percent of investigations leading to administrative actions. In fiscal year 2016, 38 percent of FPS-initiated investigations resulted in administrative actions, which did not meet the agency's fiscal year goal of 45 percent.

FPS Denies Payments Based on Medicare Rules or Policies and Not Fraud Risk

FPS prepayment edits screen individual claims to automatically deny payments that violate Medicare rules or policies. For example, some FPS edits deny claims that exceed coverage utilization limits for a service. FPS edits do not analyze individual claims to automatically deny payments

---

[15] CMS developed this measure in response to a prior GAO recommendation that the agency develop outcome-based performance goals to measure FPS's performance. See GAO-13-104.

based on risk alone or the likelihood that they are fraudulent.[16] According to CMS officials, the agency does not have the authority to use FPS to automatically deny individual claims based on risk without further evidence confirming that the claims are potentially fraudulent.[17]

Although the prepayment edits in FPS are functionally similar to those in CMS's claims processing systems, the FPS edits specifically target payments associated with potential fraud schemes. Like edits executed elsewhere in the claims processing systems, FPS edits deny payments based on rules or policies. Unlike the edits in the claims processing systems, all of the edits in FPS are designed to address identified payment vulnerabilities associated with potential fraud, according to CMS officials. Payment vulnerabilities are service- or system-specific weaknesses that can lead to improper payments, including improper payments that may be due to fraud. For example, CMS implemented an FPS edit that denies physician claims that improperly increase payments by misidentifying the location that the service was rendered. The payments are denied based on the rule that physician claims must correctly identify the place of service. The edit helped address a payment vulnerability identified by HHS OIG that found millions of dollars in overpayments.[18]

According to CMS officials, the advantage of using FPS to implement prepayment edits is that the system allows CMS to prioritize edits intended

---

[16] We previously analyzed the use of analytic systems by health care payers and did not identify any payers that use analytic systems to automatically deny individual claims based on the likelihood that they are fraudulent. See GAO-13-104.

[17] CMS may suspend payment based on reliable information of an overpayment, or pending an investigation of a credible allegation of fraud as determined in consultation with HHS OIG. 42 U.S.C. § 1395y(o); 42 C.F.R. § 405.371 (2016). CMS program integrity activities intended to address fraud generally do not focus on reviewing whether individual payments are potentially fraudulent, but instead focus on identifying suspect billing patterns and taking action against providers engaged in potential fraud. Payment denials of potentially fraudulent claims generally stem from investigations into or corrective actions taken against providers, such as payments denied for providers subject to prepayment review.

[18] Medicare payments to physicians account for overhead expenses. HHS OIG found physician claims for services performed at facility locations, such as ambulatory surgical centers, that were billed as if they had been performed at physician offices. This resulted in overpayments to physicians for office overhead expenses. See Department of Health and Human Services Office of Inspector General, *Incorrect Place-of-Service Claims Resulted in Potential Medicare Overpayments Costing Millions*, A-01-13-00506 (Washington, D.C.: May 2015).

to address payment vulnerabilities associated with potential fraud. Because CPI maintains FPS, CMS can quickly implement edits into FPS. In contrast, edits that are implemented in the claims processing systems are queued as part of quarterly system updates, and may need to compete with other claims processing system updates. CPI is not subject to such limitations when implementing edits in FPS, and officials said that edits can be developed and implemented in FPS more quickly compared to the claims processing systems.

As of May 2017, CMS had implemented 24 edits in FPS. CMS reported that in fiscal year 2015, FPS edits denied nearly 169,000 claims and saved $11.3 million. In fiscal year 2016, the edits denied nearly 324,000 claims and saved $20.4 million.[19] CMS officials stated that the number of prepayment edits implemented in FPS thus far has been limited, but that the agency is taking steps to address certain challenges that would allow the agency to develop and implement edits more quickly. For example, because of their role and expertise in processing claims, the MACs advise CPI and help develop and test FPS edits before they are implemented in the system to ensure they will work as intended. However, CPI has been limited in the amount of MAC resources that it can engage to help develop FPS edits under existing contracts. According to officials, CPI is planning to take steps to more directly involve the MACs in FPS edit development, which officials said should accelerate the edit implementation process. Additionally, CMS officials said that they plan to utilize FPS functionality to implement new edits by expanding existing edits to apply to other services. All of the 24 current FPS edits were developed from the ground up, a time and resource consuming process, according to CMS officials. In contrast, developing new edits by expanding existing edits will allow CMS to more quickly develop and implement new edits.

---

[19] As of the end of fiscal year 2016, CMS had implemented 17 edits, and officials told us that 7 additional edits have since been added. CMS reported that in fiscal year 2015, FPS edits denied $17.5 million and, in fiscal year 2016, denied $33.6 million. The savings data above excludes payments associated with denied claims that were later corrected, resubmitted, and paid, and amounts associated with resubmitted claims that were again denied by FPS.

PARTICIPANTS REPORTED THAT HFPP EFFORTS FURTHERED THEIR ABILITY TO ADDRESS HEALTH CARE FRAUD

Participants Reported That Information Sharing through HFPP Furthered Efforts to Address Fraud

HFPP participants we interviewed, including CMS officials, reported that sharing data and information within HFPP has been useful to their efforts to address health care fraud. The principal activity of HFPP is generating studies that pool and analyze multiple payers' claims data to identify providers with patterns of suspect billing across multiple payers. Study topics examine known fraud vulnerabilities important to the participating payers and are selected through a collaborative process. As an example, one study used pooled data to identify providers who were cumulatively billing multiple payers for more services than could reasonably be rendered in a single day. In another study, HFPP pooled payer information on billing codes that are frequently misused by providers engaged in potential fraud, such as codes commonly used to misrepresent non-covered services as covered. See Table 4 for a description of HFPP's completed studies as of May 2017.

Participants reported that HFPP's studies helped them to identify and take action against potentially fraudulent providers that would otherwise have gone unidentified. For instance, both public and private payers reported that HFPP's non-operational providers report uncovered providers that they had not previously identified as suspect. CMS officials and one private payer we interviewed said that they used information from this study to conduct site visits of reportedly non-operational providers. CMS officials told us that they revoked a number of the providers after confirming that they were indeed non-operational. CMS officials also said that they review the results of HFPP studies and provide information on potentially fraudulent providers to ZPICs when appropriate. The information may either serve as new leads or help support existing investigations.

Table 4. Healthcare Fraud Prevention Partnership Completed Studies as of May 2017

Study	Description
Misused Codes and Fraud Schemes	A pooled list of approximately 1400 misused codes and 100 fraud schemes.
Non-Operational Providers	A pooled list of providers that have been found to be non-operational, such as false store fronts, and only exist on paper to file claims for services that were never rendered.
Revoked/Terminated Providers	A pooled list of provider organizations that have been revoked or terminated by payers for reasons relating to fraud, waste, and abuse.
Top Billing Pharmacies for Controlled Prescription Drugs	An analysis identifying the billing pharmacies with extreme outlier dispensing of controlled prescription drugs.
Urine Drug and Genetic Testing Referrals	An analysis identifying providers with unusual referral patterns for urine drug and genetic testing.
Psycho-Therapy Timed Code Analysis	An analysis of behavioral health providers identifying those who may be cumulatively billing multiple payers for more services than could reasonably be rendered in a single day.

Source: GAO analysis of CMS information. | GAO-17-710.

Participants also reported that study results have helped them uncover payment vulnerabilities of which they might not otherwise have been aware. For example, CMS officials stated that they used the HFFP report on misused procedure codes to evaluate several Medicare payment vulnerabilities and then implemented edits to address them. In instances where participants reported that HFPP studies revealed suspect providers or schemes that were known to them, participants stated that HFPP study results helped them to confirm suspicions, better assess potential exposure, and prioritize and develop internal investigations.

Several participants we interviewed noted that even though HFPP study results can help them identify suspect providers, they may still face challenges using the information to take corrective actions. HFPP participation rules require payers to examine their internal data and claims to investigate and build cases against suspect providers before taking any corrective actions, partly in order to minimize the risk of payers taking action on false positive study results. For certain types of fraud schemes, however, the participants' internal information alone may not provide enough evidence of improper billing. For instance, although an HFPP study may reveal clear evidence that a provider is billing multiple payers for an unreasonable number of services in a single day, the provider may have only billed individual payers for a limited, reasonable number of services.

Participants reported that HFPP has also facilitated both formal and informal information sharing among payers, and indicated that it has helped them learn about fraud vulnerabilities and strategies for effectively addressing them. Formal information sharing includes presentations at HFPP meetings and a whitepaper on how payers can help address beneficiary opioid abuse and reduce opioid-related fraud.[20] HFPP also manages a web portal where participants can share individual best practices and post "fraud alerts" about emerging fraud schemes or suspect providers. Informal information sharing includes knowledge exchanged through the networking and collaboration that occurs among HFPP participants, both at in-person HFPP meetings and through collaboration that occurs via the web portal's participant directory.

HFPP Addressed Initial Data Sharing Concerns and Is Pursuing a New Data Sharing Strategy to Further Participants' Ability to Address Fraud

Although HFPP began operations in 2012, participants we interviewed stated that much of the initial work of the partnership involved negotiating the logistics for collecting and storing participants' claims data. CMS contracts with a trusted third party (TTP) entity to administer HFPP. The TTP consolidates, secures, and confidentially maintains the claims data shared by participants, and conducts studies that analyze the pooled data to identify potential fraud across payers. According to several participants we interviewed, some payers were initially reluctant to share claims data with

---

[20] See HFPP and NORC, *Healthcare Payer Strategies to Reduce the Harms of Opioids*, (January 2017), accessed February 6, 2017, https://downloads.cms.gov/files/hfpp/hfppopioid-white-paper.pdf.

the TTP because claims contain sensitive provider and beneficiary information and private payers may view them as proprietary. Accordingly, it took time for the TTP to demonstrate to payers its ability to securely store and use pooled claims data. Payers' reluctance resulted in an early time- and resource-intensive data sharing strategy that relied upon payers submitting a limited amount of claims data on a study-by-study basis, in a particular format, stripped of beneficiaries' personally identifiable information and protected health information.

Recently, HFPP began to pursue a new data sharing strategy. According to the TTP and participants we interviewed, payers will send in generalized data, reducing the data sharing burden on payers and enabling HFPP to conduct new types of studies to combat fraud. The data can be submitted in various formats, relieving payers from the need to extract and clean study-specific data. All participant data will be pooled and stored, and multiple studies will be run on the data submitted. Payers may voluntarily submit data that includes beneficiaries' personally identifiable information and protected health information. According to CMS officials, collection of personally identifiable information and protected health information will allow HFPP to conduct studies that involve identifying beneficiaries across payers, such as studies examining fraud schemes in which multiple providers fraudulently bill for the same beneficiaries.[21]

Several HFPP participants we spoke with indicated their support of the new strategy and willingness to provide beneficiaries' personally identifiable information and protected health information for more in-depth HFPP studies. As of May 2017, 38 partners had signed data sharing agreements with the new TTP. However, not all payers that previously shared claims data have agreed to participate in the new data sharing strategy and those payers are still working with the TTP to formalize agreements regarding how their claims data will be stored and used.

---

[21] CMS officials stated that beneficiary data will be de-identified by assigning beneficiaries HFPP-specific identification numbers. The de-identified beneficiary data will be stored for a period of time appropriate to conduct multiple studies.

Agency Comments

GAO provided a draft of this report to HHS. HHS provided technical comments, which GAO incorporated as appropriate.

As agreed with your offices, unless you publicly announce the contents of this report earlier, we plan no further distribution until 30 days from the report date. At that time, we will send copies to the Secretary of Health and Human Services, the Administrator of CMS, appropriate congressional requesters, and other interested parties. In addition, the report will be available at no charge on the GAO website at http://www.gao.gov.

If you or your staff members have any questions about this report, please contact me at (202) 512-7114 or at kingk@gao.gov. Contact points for our Offices of Congressional Relations and Public Affairs may be found on the last page of this report. GAO staff that made key contributions to this report are listed in appendix I.

Kathleen M. King
Director, Health Care

List of Requesters

The Honorable Greg Walden
Chairman
The Honorable Frank Pallone
Ranking Member
Committee on Energy and Commerce
House of Representatives

The Honorable Kevin Brady
Chairman
Committee on Ways and Means
House of Representatives

The Honorable Michael C. Burgess
Chairman
The Honorable Gene Green
Ranking Member
Subcommittee on Health
Committee on Energy and Commerce
House of Representatives

The Honorable Tim Murphy
Chairman
The Honorable Diana DeGette
Ranking Member
Subcommittee on Oversight and Investigations
Committee on Energy and Commerce
House of Representatives

The Honorable Patrick J. Tiberi
Chairman
The Honorable Sander Levin
Ranking Member
Subcommittee on Health
Committee on Ways and Means
House of Representatives

The Honorable Vern Buchanan
Chairman
The Honorable John Lewis
Ranking Member
Subcommittee on Oversight
Committee on Ways and Means
House of Representatives

The Honorable Peter Roskam
House of Representatives

United States Government Accountability Office

The Honorable Fred Upton
House of Representatives

APPENDIX I: GAO CONTACT AND STAFF ACKNOWLEDGMENTS

GAO Contact

Kathleen M. King, (202) 512-7114, kingk@gao.gov

Staff Acknowledgments

In addition to the contact named above, Martin T. Gahart (Assistant Director), Michael Erhardt (Analyst-in-Charge), Muriel Brown, Cathleen Hamann, Colbie Holderness, and Jennifer Whitworth made key contributions to this report.

In: Medicare: Financing, Insolvency and Fraud ISBN: 978-1-53614-811-4
Editor: Bradford Rodgers   © 2019 Nova Science Publishers, Inc.

Chapter 6

MEDICARE: ACTIONS NEEDED TO BETTER MANAGE FRAUD RISKS[*]

Seto J. Bagdoyan

WHY GAO DID THIS STUDY

Medicare covered over 58 million people in 2017 and has wide-ranging impact on the health-care sector and the overall U.S. economy. However, the billions of dollars in Medicare outlays as well as program complexity make it susceptible to improper payments, including fraud. Although there are no reliable estimates of fraud in Medicare, in fiscal year 2017 improper payments for Medicare were estimated at about $52 billion. Further, about $1.4 billion was returned to Medicare Trust Funds in fiscal year 2017 as a result of recoveries, fines, and asset forfeitures.

In December 2017, GAO issued a report examining how CMS managed its fraud risks overall and particularly the extent to which its

---

[*] This is an edited, reformatted and augmented version of United States Government Accountability Office Testimony before the Subcommittee on Oversight, Committee on Ways and Means, House of Representatives, Accessible Version, Publication No. GAO-18-660T, dated Tuesday, July 17, 2018.

efforts in the Medicare and Medicaid programs aligned with GAO's Framework. This testimony, based on that report, discusses the extent to which CMS's management of fraud risks in Medicare aligns with the Framework. For the report, GAO reviewed CMS policies and interviewed officials and external stakeholders.

WHAT GAO RECOMMENDS

In its December 2017 report, GAO made three recommendations, namely that CMS (1) require and provide fraud-awareness training to its employees; (2) conduct fraud risk assessments; and (3) create an antifraud strategy for Medicare, including an approach for evaluation. The Department of Health and Human Services agreed with these recommendations and reportedly is evaluating options to implement them. Accordingly, the recommendations remain open.

WHAT GAO FOUND

In its December 2017 report, GAO found that the Centers for Medicare & Medicaid Services' (CMS) antifraud efforts for Medicare partially align with GAO's 2015 *A Framework for Managing Fraud Risks in Federal Programs* (Framework). The Fraud Reduction and Data Analytics Act of 2015 required OMB to incorporate leading practices identified in this Framework in its guidance to agencies on addressing fraud risks.

Fraud Risk Framework's Components

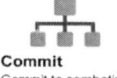

Commit
Commit to combating fraud by creating an organizational culture and structure conducive to fraud risk management.

Assess
Plan regular fraud risk assessments and assess risks to determine a fraud risk profile.

Design and Implement
Design and implement a strategy with specific control activities to mitigate assessed fraud risks and collaborate to help ensure effective implementation.

Evaluate and Adapt
Evaluate outcomes using a risk-based approach and adapt activities to improve fraud risk management.

Source: GAO. | GAO-18-660T

Medicare: Actions Needed to Better Manage Fraud Risks 147

- Consistent with the Framework, GAO determined that CMS had demonstrated commitment to combating fraud by creating a dedicated entity to lead antifraud efforts; the Center for Program Integrity (CPI) serves as this entity for fraud, waste, and abuse issues in Medicare. CMS also promoted an antifraud culture by, for example, coordinating with internal stakeholders to incorporate antifraud features into new program design. To increase awareness of fraud risks in Medicare, CMS offered and required training for stakeholder groups such as providers of medical services, but it did not offer or require similar fraud-awareness training for most of its workforce.

- CMS took some steps to identify fraud risks in Medicare; however, it had not conducted a fraud risk assessment or designed and implemented a risk-based antifraud strategy for Medicare as defined in the Framework. CMS identified fraud risks through control activities that target areas the agency designated as higher risk within Medicare, including specific provider types, such as home health agencies. Building on earlier steps and conducting a fraud risk assessment, consistent with the Framework, would provide the detailed information and insights needed to create a fraud risk profile, which, in turn, is the basis for creating an antifraud strategy.

- CMS established monitoring and evaluation mechanisms for its program-integrity control activities that, if aligned with an antifraud strategy, could enhance the effectiveness of fraud risk management in Medicare. For example, CMS used return-on-investment and savings estimates to measure the effectiveness of its Medicare program-integrity activities. In developing an antifraud strategy, consistent with the Framework, CMS could include plans for refining and building on existing methods such as return-on-investment, to evaluate the effectiveness of all of its antifraud efforts.

Chairman Jenkins, Ranking Member Lewis, and Members of the Subcommittee:

I am pleased to appear before you today to discuss ways to better manage Medicare fraud risks that we identified in a recent report.[1] Although there are no reliable estimates of fraud in Medicare, in fiscal year 2017 improper payments for Medicare were estimated at about $52 billion.[2]

A recent example illustrates the scope and scale of fraud risks. The Department of Health and Human Services (HHS) Office of Inspector General's (OIG) latest Semiannual Report to Congress highlighted the recent activities of the Medicare Fraud Strike Force (Strike Force).[3] During the period from October 1, 2017, through March 31, 2018, Strike Force efforts resulted in the filing of charges against 77 individuals or entities, 107 criminal actions, and more than $100.3 million in investigative receivables. In one example, a Strike Force investigation led to the conviction of two owners of a medical billing company, who were both found guilty of conspiracy and health-care fraud, for fraudulently billing Medicare for services that were never provided. They also conspired to circumvent Medicare's fraud investigation of one of the owners by creating sham companies. The owners were sentenced to 10 years in prison, and 15 years in prison, respectively, and ordered to pay nearly $9.2 million in restitution.

---

[1] GAO, Medicare and Medicaid: CMS Needs to Fully Align Its Antifraud Efforts with the Fraud Risk Framework, GAO-18-88 (Washington, D.C.: Dec. 5, 2017).

[2] An improper payment is defined as any payment that should not have been made or that was made in an incorrect amount (including overpayments and underpayments) under statutory, contractual, administrative, or other legally applicable requirements. It includes any payment to an ineligible recipient, any payment for an ineligible good or service, any duplicate payment, any payment for a good or service not received (except for such payments where authorized by law), and any payment that does not account for credit for applicable discounts. See 31 U.S.C. § 3321 note. OMB guidance also instructs agencies to report as improper payments any payment for which insufficient or no documentation was found.

[3] Medicare Fraud Strike Force, a joint Department of Justice (DOJ) and HHS OIG program, consists of investigators and prosecutors who use data-analysis and traditional law-enforcement techniques to identify, investigate, and prosecute potentially fraudulent billing patterns in geographic areas with high rates of health-care fraud.

Overall, HHS OIG and the Department of Justice report annually on monetary and other results of their efforts against health-care fraud and abuse: in fiscal year 2017, about $1.4 billion was returned to Medicare Trust Funds as a result of recoveries, fines, and asset forfeitures.[4]

Medicare, which is administered within HHS by its Centers for Medicare & Medicaid Services (CMS), has been on our high-risk list since 1990[5] because of the size and complexity of the program, and its susceptibility to fraud, waste, and abuse. Medicare covered over 58 million people in 2017 and it has wide-ranging current and long-term effects beyond beneficiaries, the health-care sector, and the overall U.S. economy. The following statistics illustrate the program's impact.

- According to the Congressional Budget Office (CBO), in 2017 Medicare outlays totaled $702 billion. Under current law, the outlays are projected to rise to $1.5 trillion in 2028, growing at about 7 percent a year; that is, faster than the economy, as the population ages and health-care costs rise.[6]
- In 2017, these expenditures accounted for 3.7 percent of gross domestic product (GDP) and 17.6 percent of federal outlays. CBO estimates that, in 2028, under current law, Medicare will account for 5.1 percent of GDP and 21.9 percent of federal outlays.
- Over 1 million health-care providers, contractors, and suppliers from across the health sector—including private health plans, physicians, hospitals, skilled-nursing facilities, durable medical equipment suppliers, ambulance providers, and many others—receive payments from Medicare.

Given the size and impact of Medicare on the health-care sector and U.S. economy overall, we recently reported on CMS's fraud risk

---

[4] Department of Health and Human Services and Department of Justice, Health Care Fraud and Abuse Control Program: Annual Report for Fiscal Year 2017.

[5] GAO, High-Risk Series: Progress on Many High-Risk Areas, While Substantial Efforts Needed on Others, GAO-17-317 (Washington, D.C.: Feb. 15, 2017).

[6] Congressional Budget Office, The Budget and Economic Outlook: 2018 to 2028 (April 2018).

management efforts relative to GAO's 2015 *A Framework for Managing Fraud Risks in Federal Programs* (Fraud Risk Framework).[7] The Fraud Risk Framework describes key components and leading practices for agencies to proactively and strategically manage fraud risks. Our objectives in the December 2017 report were to determine: (1) CMS's approach for managing fraud risks across its four principal programs (including Medicare) and (2) how CMS's efforts for managing fraud risks in Medicare and Medicaid align with the Fraud Risk Framework.

Drawing from the December 2017 report, my testimony today discusses the extent to which CMS's management of fraud risks in Medicare aligned with the Fraud Risk Framework and the actions needed to better manage fraud risks.

We performed our work on CMS antifraud efforts in Medicare and Medicaid for the December 2017 report under the authority of the Comptroller General to assist Congress with its oversight. The report provides further detail on our scope and methodology. Because this statement focuses on Medicare, we have omitted references to Medicaid in some instances when discussing organizational structure and agency-wide efforts.

We conducted the work in the December 2017 report in accordance with generally accepted government auditing standards. Those standards require that we plan and perform the audit to obtain sufficient, appropriate evidence to provide a reasonable basis for our findings and conclusions based on our audit objectives. We believe that the evidence obtained provides a reasonable basis for our findings and conclusions based on our audit objectives.

---

[7] GAO, A Framework for Managing Fraud Risks in Federal Programs, GAO-15-593SP (Washington, D.C.: July 2015).

BACKGROUND

Medicare is one of four principal health-insurance programs administered by CMS; it provides health insurance for persons aged 65 and over, certain individuals with disabilities, and individuals with end-stage renal disease.[8] See table 1 for information about Medicare's component programs.

Table 1. Summary of Medicare Parts

Medicare program	Program description
Medicare Fee-for-Service (FFS) (Parts A and B)	Providers submit claims for reimbursement after services have been rendered. Medicare pays providers for each service delivered (e.g., office visit, test, or procedure). Part A—hospital insurance Part B—outpatient care
Medicare Advantage (Part C)	Alternative to Parts A and B that allows beneficiaries to receive Medicare benefits through a private health plan[a]
Medicare Prescription Drug (Part D)	Voluntary, outpatient prescription-drug coverage through stand-alone drug plans or Medicare Advantage drug plans

Source: GAO. | GAO-18-660T.

[a] Health-insurance plans are paid a predetermined, fixed periodic amount per enrollee. The payment is risk-adjusted based on enrollee diagnoses, but that does not vary based on number or cost of health-care services an enrollee uses.

Medicare is the largest CMS program, at $702 billion in fiscal year 2017. As discussed earlier, according to CBO, Medicare outlays are projected to rise to $1.5 trillion in 2028 (see figure 1).

---

[8] Other CMS programs are Medicaid, the Children's Health Insurance Program (CHIP), and the health-insurance marketplaces.

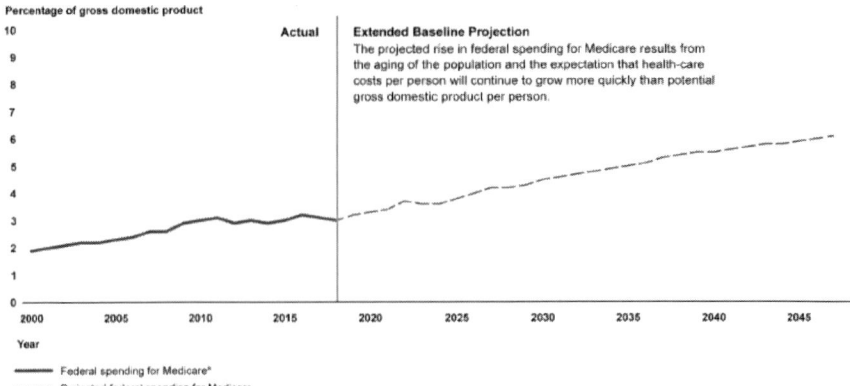

Source: Congressional Budget Office (CBO).| GAO-18-660T.

a Spending for Medicare refers to net spending for Medicare, which accounts for offsetting receipts that are credited to the program. Those offsetting receipts are mostly premium payments made by beneficiaries to the government.

Figure 1. Federal Spending on Medicare Is Projected to Increase.

Data Table for Figure 1: Federal Spending on Medicare Is Projected to Increase

n/a	Percentage of gross domestic product
Year	Medicare
2000	1.9
2001	2
2002	2.1
2003	2.2
2004	2.2
2005	2.3
2006	2.4
2007	2.6
2008	2.6
2009	2.9
2010	3
2011	3.1
2012	2.9
2013	3

Medicare: Actions Needed to Better Manage Fraud Risks 153

n/a	Percentage of gross domestic product
Year	Medicare
2014	2.9
2015	3
2016	3.2
2017	3.1
2018	3
2019	3.2
2020	3.3
2021	3.4
2022	3.7
2023	3.6
2024	3.6
2025	3.8
2026	4
2027	4.2
2028	4.2
2029	4.3
2030	4.5
2031	4.6
2032	4.7
2033	4.8
2034	4.9
2035	5
2036	5.1
2037	5.3
2038	5.4
2039	5.5
2040	5.5
2041	5.6
2042	5.7
2043	5.8
2044	5.8
2045	5.9
2046	6
2047	6.1

Fraud Vulnerabilities and Improper Payments in Medicare

Fraud involves obtaining something of value through willful misrepresentation. There are no reliable estimates of the extent of fraud in the Medicare program, or in the health-care industry as a whole. By its very nature, fraud is difficult to detect, as those involved are engaged in intentional deception. Further, potential fraud cases must be identified, investigated, prosecuted, and adjudicated—resulting in a conviction—before fraud can be established.

As I mentioned earlier, we designated Medicare as a high-risk program in 1990 because its size, scope, and complexity make it vulnerable to fraud, waste, and abuse. Similarly, the Office of Management and Budget (OMB) designated all parts of Medicare a "high priority" program because they each report $750 million or more in improper payments in a given year.[9] We also highlighted challenges associated with duplicative payments in Medicare in our annual report on duplication and opportunities for cost savings in federal programs.[10]

Improper payments are a significant risk to the Medicare program and may include payments made as a result of fraud. However, I would note that improper payments are not a proxy for the amount of fraud or extent of fraud risk in a particular program as improper payment measurement does not specifically identify or estimate such payments due to fraud. Improper payments are those that are either made in an incorrect amount (overpayments and underpayments) or those that should not have been made at all.

---

[9] Starting in fiscal year 2018, the threshold for high-priority program determinations is $2 billion in improper payments regardless of the improper payment rate.

[10] GAO, 2017 Annual Report: Additional Opportunities to Reduce Fragmentation, Overlap, and Duplication and Achieve Other Financial Benefits, GAO-17-491SP (Washington, D.C.: April 2017).

CMS's Fraud Risk Management Approach

Our December 2017 report found that CMS manages its fraud risks as part of a broader program-integrity approach working with a broad array of stakeholders. CMS's program-integrity approach includes efforts to address waste, abuse, and improper payments as well as fraud across its four principal programs. In Medicare, CMS collaborates with contractors, health-insurance plans, and law-enforcement and other agencies to carry out its program-integrity responsibilities. According to CMS officials, this broader program-integrity approach can help the agency develop control activities to address multiple sources of improper payments, including fraud.

Fraud Risk Management Standards and Guidance

According to federal standards and guidance, executive-branch agency managers are responsible for managing fraud risks and implementing practices for combating those risks. Federal internal control standards call for agency management officials to assess the internal and external risks their entities face as they seek to achieve their objectives. The standards state that as part of this overall assessment, management should consider the potential for fraud when identifying, analyzing, and responding to risks.[11] Risk management is a formal and disciplined practice for addressing risk and reducing it to an acceptable level.[12]

In July 2015, GAO issued the Fraud Risk Framework, which provides a comprehensive set of key components and leading practices that serve as a guide for agency managers to use when developing efforts to combat fraud in a strategic, risk-based way.[13] The Fraud Risk Framework describes

---

[11] GAO, *Standards for Internal Control in the Federal Government*, GAO-14-704G (Washington, D.C.: September 2014).

[12] MITRE, *Government-wide Payment Integrity: New approaches and Solutions Needed* (McLean, Va.: February 2016).

[13] See GAO-15-593SP.

leading practices in four components: commit, assess, design and implement, and evaluate and adapt, as depicted in figure 2.

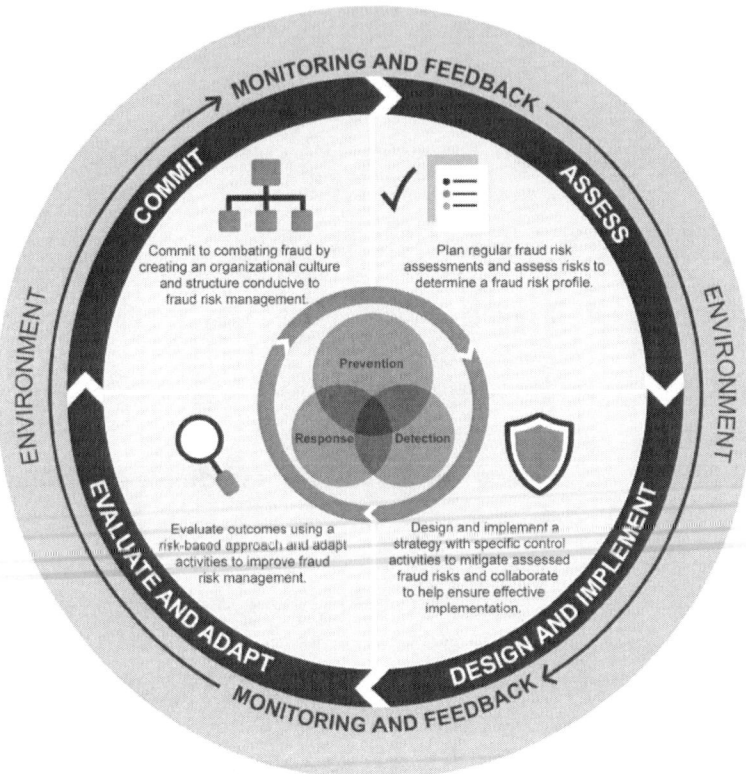

Source: GAO-18-660T.

Figure 2. The Fraud Risk Management Framework.

The Fraud Reduction and Data Analytics Act of 2015, enacted in June 2016, requires OMB to establish guidelines for federal agencies to create controls to identify and assess fraud risks and design and implement antifraud control activities. The act further requires OMB to incorporate the leading practices from the Fraud Risk Framework in the guidelines. In July 2016, OMB published guidance about enterprise risk management and internal controls in federal executive departments and agencies.[14] Among

---

[14] Office of Management and Budget, *Management's Responsibility for Enterprise Risk Management and Internal Control*, Circular No. A-123 (Washington, D.C.: July 15, 2016).

other things, this guidance affirms that managers should adhere to the leading practices identified in the Fraud Risk Framework. Further, the act requires federal agencies to submit to Congress a progress report each year for 3 consecutive years on the implementation of the controls established under OMB guidelines, among other things.[15]

CMS's EFFORTS MANAGING FRAUD RISKS IN MEDICARE WERE PARTIALLY ALIGNED WITH THE FRAUD RISK FRAMEWORK

CMS's antifraud efforts partially aligned with the Fraud Risk Framework. Consistent with the framework, CMS has demonstrated commitment to combating fraud by creating a dedicated entity to lead antifraud efforts. It has also taken steps to establish a culture conducive to fraud risk management, although it could expand its antifraud training to include all employees. CMS has taken some steps to identify fraud risks in Medicare; however, it has not conducted a fraud risk assessment or developed a risk-based antifraud strategy for Medicare as defined in the Fraud Risk Framework. CMS has established monitoring and evaluation mechanisms for its program-integrity control activities that, if aligned with a risk-based antifraud strategy, could enhance the effectiveness of fraud risk management in Medicare.

CMS's Organizational Structure Includes a Dedicated Entity for Program-Integrity and Antifraud Efforts

The *commit* component of the Fraud Risk Framework calls for an agency to commit to combating fraud by creating an organizational culture and structure conducive to fraud risk management. This component

---

[15] Pub. L. No. 114-186, § 3, 130 Stat. 546 (2016).

includes establishing a dedicated entity to lead fraud risk management activities.[16]

Within CMS, the Center for Program Integrity (CPI) serves as the dedicated entity for fraud, waste, and abuse issues in Medicare, which is consistent with the Fraud Risk Framework. CPI was established in 2010, in response to a November 2009 Executive Order on reducing improper payments and eliminating waste in federal programs.[17] This formalized role, according to CMS officials, elevated the status of program-integrity efforts, which previously were carried out by other parts of CMS.

As an executive-level Center—on the same level with five other executive-level Centers at CMS, such as the Center for Medicare—CPI has a direct reporting line to executive-level management at CMS. The Fraud Risk Framework identifies a direct reporting line to senior-level managers within the agency as a leading practice. According to CMS officials, this elevated organizational status offers CPI heightened visibility across CMS, attention by CMS executive leadership, and involvement in executive-level conversations.

CMS Has Taken Steps to Create a Culture Conducive to Fraud Risk Management but Could Enhance Antifraud Training for Employees

The *commit* component of the Fraud Risk Framework also includes creating an organizational culture to combat fraud at all levels of the agency. Consistent with the Fraud Risk Framework, CMS has promoted an antifraud culture by, for example, coordinating with internal and external stakeholders.

Consistent with leading practices in the Fraud Risk Framework to involve all levels of the agency in setting an antifraud tone, CPI has worked collaboratively with other CMS Centers. In addition to engaging

---

[16] See GAO-15-593SP.

[17] Reducing Improper Payments, Exec. Order No. 13520, 74 Fed. Reg. 226 (Nov. 20, 2009).

executive-level officials of other CMS Centers through the Program Integrity Board, CPI has worked collaboratively with other Centers within CMS to incorporate antifraud features into new program design or policy development and established regular communication at the staff level. For example:

- Center for Medicare and Medicaid Innovation (CMMI). When developing the Medicare Diabetes Prevention Program, CMMI officials told us they worked with CPI's Provider Enrollment and Oversight Group and Governance Management Group to develop risk-based screening procedures for entities that would enroll in Medicare to provide diabetes-prevention services, among other activities. The program was expanded nationally in 2016, and CMS determined that an entity may enroll in Medicare as a program supplier if it satisfies enrollment requirements, including that the supplier must pass existing high categorical risk-level screening requirements.[18]
- Center for Medicare (CM). In addition to building safeguards into programs and developing policies, CM officials told us that there are several standing meetings, on monthly, biweekly, and weekly bases, between groups within CM and CPI that discuss issues related to provider enrollment, FFS operations, and contractor management. A senior CM official also told us that there are ad hoc meetings taking place between CM and CPI: "We interact multiple times daily at different levels of the organization. Working closely is just a regular part of our business."

CMS has also demonstrated its commitment to addressing fraud, waste, and abuse to its stakeholders. Representatives of CMS's extensive stakeholder network whom we interviewed—contractors and officials from

---

[18] 82 Fed. Reg. 52,976 (Nov. 15, 2017) (codified at 42 C.F.R. Parts 405, 410, 414, 424, and 425). For additional information about CMS provider-enrollment activities for Medicare, see GAO, *Medicare: Initial Results of Revised Process to Screen Providers and Suppliers, and Need for Objectives and Performance Measures*, GAO-17-42 (Washington, D.C.: Nov. 15, 2016).

public and private entities—generally recognized the agency's commitment to combating fraud. In our interviews with stakeholders, officials observed CMS's increased commitment over time to address fraud, waste, and abuse and cited examples of specific CMS actions. CMS contractors told us that CMS's commitment to combating fraud is incorporated into contractual requirements, such as requiring (1) data analysis for potential fraud leads and (2) fraud-awareness training for providers. Officials from entities that are members of the Healthcare Fraud Prevention Partnership (HFPP), specifically, a health-insurance plan and the National Health Care Anti-Fraud Association, added that CMS's effort to establish the HFPP and its ongoing collaboration and information sharing reflect CMS's commitment to combat fraud in Medicare.[19]

The Fraud Risk Framework identifies training as one way of demonstrating an agency's commitment to combating fraud. Training and education intended to increase fraud awareness among stakeholders, managers, and employees serve as a preventive measure to help create a culture of integrity and compliance within the agency. The Fraud Risk Framework discusses requiring all employees to attend training upon hiring and on an ongoing basis thereafter.

To increase awareness of fraud risks in Medicare, CMS offers and requires training for stakeholder groups such as providers, beneficiaries, and health-insurance plans. Specifically, through its National Training Program and Medicare Learning Network, CMS makes available training materials on combating Medicare fraud, waste, and abuse.[20] These materials help to identify and report fraud, waste, and abuse in CMS programs and are geared toward providers, beneficiaries, as well as trainers

---

[19] In 2012, CMS created the HFPP to share information with public and private stakeholders and to conduct studies related to health-care fraud, waste, and abuse. According to CMS, as of October 2017, the HFPP included 89 public and private partners, including Medicare- and Medicaid-related federal and state agencies, law-enforcement agencies, private health-insurance plans, and antifraud and other health-care organizations.

[20] The CMS National Training Program provides support for partners and stakeholders, not-for-profit professionals and volunteers who work with seniors and people with disabilities, and others who help people make informed health-care decisions. The program offers an online training library with materials to conduct outreach and education sessions. The Medicare Learning Network provides free educational materials for healthcare professionals on CMS programs, policies, and initiatives.

and other stakeholders. Separately, CMS requires health-insurance plans working with CMS to provide annual fraud, waste, and abuse training to their employees.[21]

However, CMS does not offer or require similar fraud-awareness training for the majority of its workforce. For a relatively small portion of its overall workforce—specifically, contracting officer representatives who are responsible for certain aspects of the acquisition function—CMS requires completion of fraud and abuse prevention training every 2 years. According to CMS, 638 of its contracting officer representatives (or about 10 percent of its overall workforce) completed such training in 2016 and 2017. Although CMS offers fraud-awareness training to others, the agency does not require fraud-awareness training for new hires or on a regular basis for all employees because the agency has focused on providing process-based internal controls training for its employees.

While fraud-awareness training for contracting officer representatives is an important step in helping to promote fraud risk management, fraud-awareness training specific to CMS programs would be beneficial for all employees. Such training would not only be consistent with what CMS offers to or requires of its stakeholders and some of its employees, but would also help to keep the agency's entire workforce continuously aware of fraud risks and examples of known fraud schemes, such as those identified in successful HHS OIG investigations. Such training would also keep employees informed as they administer CMS programs or develop agency policies and procedures. Considering the vulnerability of Medicare and Medicaid programs to fraud, waste, and abuse, without regular required training CMS cannot be assured that its workforce of over 6,000 employees is continuously aware of risks facing its programs.

In our December 2017 report, we recommended that the Administrator of CMS provide fraud-awareness training relevant to risks facing CMS programs and require new hires to undergo such training and all employees to undergo training on a recurring basis. In its March 2018 letter to GAO, HHS stated that CMS is in the process of developing Fraud, Waste, and

---

[21] For example, 42 C.F.R. § 422.503(b)(4)(vi)(C).

Abuse Training for all new employees, to be presented at CMS New Employee Orientations. Additionally, CMS is also developing training to be completed by current CMS employees on an annual basis. As of July 2018, this recommendation remains open.

CMS Has Taken Steps to Identify Fraud Risks but Has Not Conducted a Fraud Risk Assessment for Medicare

The *assess* component of the Fraud Risk Framework calls for federal managers to plan regular fraud risk assessments and to assess risks to determine a fraud risk profile.[22] Identifying fraud risks is one of the steps included in the Fraud Risk Framework for assessing risks to determine a fraud risk profile.

In our December 2017 report, we discussed several examples of steps CMS has taken to identify fraud risks as well as control activities that target areas the agency has designated as higher risk within Medicare, including specific provider types and specific geographic locations. These examples include

- data analytics to assist investigations in Medicare FFS, including Medicare's Fraud Prevention System (FPS),[23]
- prior authorization for Medicare FFS services or supplies,[24]
- revised provider screening and enrollment processes for Medicare FFS,[25] and

---

[22] According to the Fraud Risk Framework, a fraud risk profile documents the findings from a fraud risk assessment. We discuss this concept later in the report.

[23] The FPS is a data-analytic system that analyzes Medicare fee-for-service claims to identify health-care providers with suspect billing patterns for further investigation and to prevent improper payments. See GAO, *Medicare: CMS Fraud Prevention System Uses Claims Analysis to Address Fraud*, GAO-17-710 (Washington, D.C.: Aug. 30, 2017).

[24] Prior authorization is a payment approach that generally requires health-care providers and suppliers to first demonstrate compliance with coverage and payment rules before certain items or services are provided to patients, rather than after the items or services have been provided. See GAO, *Medicare: CMS Should Take Actions to Continue Prior Authorization Efforts to Reduce Spending*, GAO-18-341 (Washington, D.C.: Apr. 20, 2018).

- temporary provider enrollment moratoriums for certain providers and geographic areas for Medicare FFS.

CMS officials told us that CPI initially focused on developing control activities for Medicare FFS and consider these activities to be the most mature of all CPI efforts to address fraud risks.

CMS Has Not Conducted a Fraud Risk Assessment for Medicare

The assess component of the Fraud Risk Framework calls for federal managers to plan regular fraud risk assessments and assess risks to determine a fraud risk profile. Furthermore, federal internal control standards call for agency management to assess the internal and external risks their entities face as they seek to achieve their objectives. The standards state that, as part of this overall assessment, management should consider the potential for fraud when identifying, analyzing, and responding to risks.[26]

The Fraud Risk Framework states that, in planning the fraud risk assessment, effective managers tailor the fraud risk assessment to the program by, among other things, identifying appropriate tools, methods, and sources for gathering information about fraud risks and involving relevant stakeholders in the assessment process. Fraud risk assessments that align with the Fraud Risk Framework involve (1) identifying inherent fraud risks affecting the program, (2) assessing the likelihood and impact of those fraud risks, (3) determining fraud risk tolerance, (4) examining the suitability of existing fraud controls and prioritizing residual fraud risks, and (5) documenting the results (see figure 3).

---

[25] GAO-17-42.
[26] GAO-14-704G.

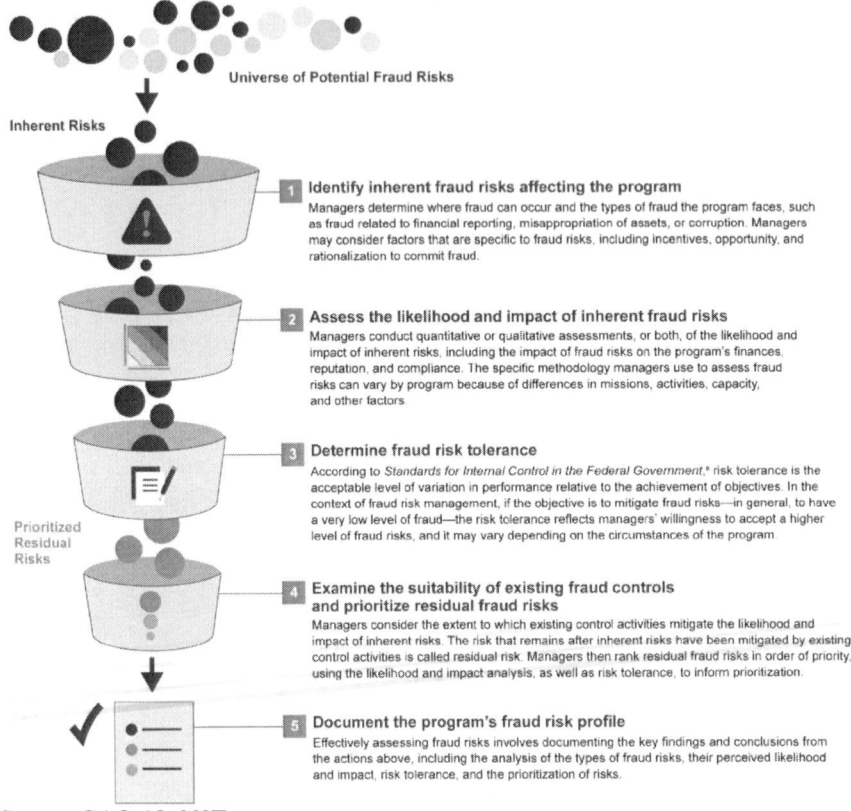

Source: GAO-18-660T.

Figure 3. Key Elements of the Fraud Risk Assessment Process.

Although CMS had identified some fraud risks posed by providers in Medicare FFS, the agency had not conducted a fraud risk assessment for the Medicare program as a whole. Such a risk assessment would provide the detailed information and insights needed to create a fraud risk profile, which, in turn, is the basis for creating an antifraud strategy.

According to CMS officials, CMS had not conducted a fraud risk assessment for Medicare because, within CPI's broader approach of preventing and eliminating improper payments, its focus has been on addressing specific vulnerabilities among provider groups that have shown themselves particularly prone to fraud, waste, and abuse. With this approach, however, it is unlikely that CMS will be able to design and

Medicare: Actions Needed to Better Manage Fraud Risks   165

implement the most-appropriate control activities to respond to the full portfolio of fraud risks.

A fraud risk assessment consists of discrete activities that build upon each other. Specifically:

- *Identifying inherent fraud risks affecting the program.* As discussed earlier, CMS took steps to identify fraud risks. However, CMS has not used a process to identify inherent fraud risks from the universe of potential vulnerabilities facing Medicare, including threats from various sources. According to CPI officials, most of the agency's fraud control activities are focused on fraud risks posed by providers. The Fraud Risk Framework discusses fully considering inherent fraud risks from internal and external sources in light of fraud risk factors such as incentives, opportunities, and rationalization to commit fraud. For example, according to CMS officials, the inherent design of the Medicare Part C program may pose fraud risks that are challenging to detect.[27] A fraud risk assessment would help CMS identify all sources of fraudulent behaviors, beyond threats posed by providers, such as those posed by health-insurance plans, contractors, or employees.

- *Assessing the likelihood and impact of fraud risks and determining fraud risk tolerance.* CMS has taken steps to prioritize fraud risks in some areas, but it had not assessed the likelihood or impact of fraud risks or determined fraud risk tolerance across all parts of Medicare. Assessing the likelihood and impact of inherent fraud risks would involve consideration of the impact of fraud risks on program finances, reputation, and compliance. Without assessing the likelihood and impact of risks in Medicare or internally determining which fraud risks may fall under the tolerance

---

[27] In Medicare Part C, health-insurance plans may pose a fraud risk, as shown by a recent legal settlement. See the Freedom Health case at Department of Justice, *Medicare Advantage Organization and Former Chief Operating Officer to Pay $32.5 Million to Settle False Claims Act Allegations*, May 30, 2017, accessed May 31, 2017, https://www.justice.gov/opa/pr/medicare-advantage-organization-and-former-chiefoperating-officer-pay-325-million-settle.

threshold, CMS cannot be certain that it is aware of the most-significant fraud risks facing this program and what risks it is willing to tolerate based on the program's size and complexity.

- *Examining the suitability of existing fraud controls and prioritizing residual fraud risks.* CMS had not assessed existing control activities or prioritized residual fraud risks. According to the Fraud Risk Framework, managers may consider the extent to which existing control activities—whether focused on prevention, detection, or response—mitigate the likelihood and impact of inherent risks and whether the remaining risks exceed managers' tolerance. This analysis would help CMS to prioritize residual risks and to determine mitigation approaches. For example, CMS had not established preventive fraud control activities in Medicare Part C. Using a fraud risk assessment for Medicare Part C and closely examining existing fraud control activities and residual risks, CMS could be better positioned to address fraud risks facing this growing program and develop preventive control activities.[28] Furthermore, without assessing existing fraud control activities and prioritizing residual fraud risks, CMS cannot be assured that its current control activities are addressing the most-significant risks. Such analysis would also help CMS determine whether additional, preferably preventive, fraud controls are needed to mitigate residual risks, make adjustments to existing control activities, and potentially scale back or remove control activities that are addressing tolerable fraud risks.

- *Documenting the risk-assessment results in a fraud risk profile.* CMS had not developed a fraud risk profile that documents key

---

[28] We have reported about concerns with improper payments in Part C. For example, we examined CMS's audits of Medicare Advantage organizations—which help CMS recover improper payments in cases where beneficiary diagnoses are unsupported by medical records—and recommended that CMS improve the timeliness of, and processes for, selecting contracts to include in its audits. We have also recommended that CMS develop specific plans for incorporating a recovery auditor into the agency's Part C audit program. Both recommendations remain open. See GAO, *Medicare Advantage Program Integrity: CMS's Efforts to Ensure Proper Payments and Identify and Recover Improper Payments*, GAO-17-761T (July 19, 2017).

findings and conclusions of the fraud risk assessment. According to the Fraud Risk Framework, the risk profile can also help agencies decide how to allocate resources to respond to residual fraud risks. Given the large size and complexity of Medicare, a documented fraud risk profile could support CMS's resource-allocation decisions as well as facilitate the transfer of knowledge and continuity across CMS staff and changing administrations.

Senior CPI officials told us that the agency plans to start a fraud risk assessment for Medicare after it completes a separate fraud risk assessment of the federally facilitated marketplace. This fraud risk assessment for the federally facilitated marketplace eligibility and enrollment process is being conducted in response to a recommendation we made in February 2016.[29] In April 2017, CPI officials told us that this fraud risk assessment was largely completed, although in September 2017 CPI officials told us that the assessment was undergoing agency review. CPI officials told us that they have informed CM officials that there will be future fraud risk assessments for Medicare; however, they could not provide estimated timelines or plans for conducting such assessments, such as the order or programmatic scope of the assessments.

Once completed, CMS could use the federally facilitated marketplace fraud risk assessment and apply any lessons learned when planning for and designing fraud risk assessments for Medicare. According to the Fraud Risk Framework, factors such as size, resources, maturity of the agency or program, and experience in managing risks can influence how the entity plans the fraud risk assessment. Additionally, effective managers tailor the fraud risk assessment to the program when planning for it. The large scale and complexity of Medicare as well as time and resources involved in conducting a fraud risk assessment underscore the importance of a well-planned and tailored approach to identifying the assessment's programmatic scope. Planning and tailoring may involve decisions to conduct a fraud risk assessment for Medicare as a whole or divided into

---

[29] GAO, Patient Protection and Affordable Care Act: CMS Should Act to Strengthen Enrollment Controls and Manage Fraud Risk, GAO-16-29 (Washington, D.C.: Feb. 23, 2016).

several sub-assessments to reflect their various component parts (e.g., Medicare Part C).

CMS's existing fraud risk identification efforts as well as communication channels with stakeholders could serve as a foundation for developing a fraud risk assessment for Medicare. The leading practices identified in the Fraud Risk Framework discuss the importance of identifying appropriate tools, methods, and sources for gathering information about fraud risks and involving relevant stakeholders in the assessment process. CMS's fraud risk identification efforts discussed earlier could provide key information about fraud risks and their likelihood and impact. Furthermore, existing relationships and communication channels across CMS and its extensive network of stakeholders could support building a comprehensive understanding of known and potential fraud risks for the purposes of a fraud risk assessment. For example, the fraud vulnerabilities identified through data analysis and information sharing with health-insurance plans, law-enforcement organizations, and contractors could inform a fraud risk assessment. CPI's Command Center missions—facilitated collaboration sessions that bring together experts from various disciplines to improve the processes for fraud prevention in Medicare[30]—could bring together experts to identify potential or emerging fraud vulnerabilities or to brainstorm approaches to mitigate residual fraud risks.

As CMS makes plans to move forward with a fraud risk assessment for Medicare, it will be important to consider the frequency with which the fraud risk assessment would need to be updated. While, according to the Fraud Risk Framework, the time intervals between updates can vary based on the programmatic and operating environment, assessing fraud risks on an ongoing basis is important to ensure that control activities are continuously addressing fraud risks. The constantly evolving fraud schemes, the size of the programs in terms of beneficiaries and

---

[30] According to CMS, the Command Center opened in July 2012 and provides an opportunity for Medicare and Medicaid policy experts, law-enforcement officials from the HHS OIG and the Federal Bureau of Investigation, clinicians, and CMS fraud investigators to collaborate before, during, and after the development of fraud leads in real time. In fiscal year 2015, CMS conducted 41 Command Center missions.

expenditures, as well as continual changes in Medicare—such as development of innovative payment models and increasing managed-care enrollment—call for constant vigilance and regular updates to the fraud risk assessment.

In our December 2017 report we recommended that the Administrator of CMS conduct fraud risk assessments for Medicare and Medicaid to include respective fraud risk profiles and plans for regularly updating the assessments and profiles. In its March 2018 letter to GAO, HHS stated that it is currently evaluating its options with regards to implementing this recommendation. As of July 2018, the recommendation remains open.

CMS Needs to Develop a Risk-Based Antifraud Strategy for Medicare, Which Would Include Plans for Monitoring and Evaluation

The *design and implement* component of the Fraud Risk Framework calls for federal managers to design and implement a strategy with specific control activities to mitigate assessed fraud risks and collaborate to help ensure effective implementation.

According to the Fraud Risk Framework, effective managers develop and document an antifraud strategy that describes the program's approach for addressing the prioritized fraud risks identified during the fraud risk assessment, also referred to as a risk-based antifraud strategy. A risk-based antifraud strategy describes existing fraud control activities as well as any new fraud control activities a program may adopt to address residual fraud risks. In developing a strategy and antifraud control activities, effective managers focus on fraud prevention over detection, develop a plan for responding to identified instances of fraud, establish collaborative relationships with stakeholders, and create incentives to help effectively implement the strategy. Additionally, as part of a documented strategy, management identifies roles and responsibilities of those involved in fraud risk management activities; describes control activities as well as plans for monitoring and evaluation; creates timelines; and communicates the antifraud strategy to employees and stakeholders, among other things.

As discussed earlier, CMS had some control activities in place to identify fraud risk in Medicare, particularly in the FFS program.[31] However, CMS had not developed and documented a risk-based antifraud strategy to guide its design and implementation of new antifraud activities and to better align and coordinate its existing activities to ensure it is targeting and mitigating the most-significant fraud risks.

Antifraud strategy. CMS officials told us that CPI does not have a documented risk-based antifraud strategy. Although CMS has developed several documents that describe efforts to address fraud,[32] the agency had not developed a risk-based antifraud strategy for Medicare because, as discussed earlier, it had not conducted a fraud risk assessment that would serve as a foundation for such strategy.

In 2016, CPI identified five strategic objectives for program integrity, which include antifraud elements and an emphasis on prevention.[33] However, according to CMS officials, these objectives were identified from discussions with CMS leadership and various stakeholders and not through a fraud risk assessment process to identify inherent fraud risks from the universe of potential vulnerabilities, as described earlier and called for in the leading practices. These strategic objectives were presented at an antifraud conference in 2016,[34] but were not announced publicly until the release of the Annual Report to Congress on the

---

[31] The individual CMS fraud control activities and other antifraud efforts described in the December 2017 report serve as examples of CMS activities; we did not evaluate the effectiveness of these efforts.

[32] Centers for Medicare & Medicaid Services, New Strategic Direction and Key Antifraud Activities (Nov. 3, 2011); Comprehensive Medicaid Integrity Plan: Fiscal Years 2014-2018; Annual Report to Congress on the Medicare and Medicaid Integrity Programs for Fiscal Year 2015; Annual Report to Congress on the Medicare and Medicaid Integrity Programs for Fiscal Years 2013 and 2014; CMS Medicare and Medicaid Program Integrity Strategy (Mar. 3, 2013).

[33] The five strategic objectives are: (1) address the full spectrum of fraud, waste, and abuse; (2) proactively manage provider screening and enrollment; (3) continue to build states' capacity to protect Medicaid; (4) extend work in Medicare Parts C and D, Medicaid managed care, and the Marketplace; and (5) provide greater transparency into program-integrity issues.

[34] National Health Care Anti-Fraud Association conference in Atlanta, Georgia, November 15–18, 2016.

Medicare and Medicaid Integrity Programs for Fiscal Year 2015 in June 2017.

Stakeholder relationships and communication. CMS has established relationships and communicated with stakeholders, but, without an antifraud strategy, stakeholders we spoke with lacked a common understanding of CMS's strategic approach. Prior work on practices that can help federal agencies collaborate effectively calls for a strategy that is shared with stakeholders to promote trust and understanding.[35] Once an antifraud strategy is developed, the Fraud Risk Framework calls for managers to collaborate to ensure effective implementation. Although some CMS stakeholders were able to describe various CMS program-integrity priorities and activities, such as home health being a fraud risk priority, the stakeholders could not communicate, articulate, or cite a common CMS strategic approach to address fraud risks in its programs.

Incentives. The Fraud Risk Framework discusses creating incentives to help ensure effective implementation of the antifraud strategy once it is developed. Currently, some incentives within stakeholder relationships may complicate CMS's antifraud efforts. Among contractors, CMS encourages information sharing through conferences and workshops; however, competition for CMS business among contractors can be a disincentive to information sharing. CMS officials acknowledged this concern and said that they expect contractors to share information related to fraud schemes, outcomes of investigations, and tips for addressing fraud, but not proprietary information such as algorithms to risk-score providers.

Without developing and documenting an antifraud strategy based on a fraud risk assessment, as called for in the *design and implement* component of the Fraud Risk Framework, CMS cannot ensure that it has a coordinated approach to address the range of fraud risks and to appropriately target and allocate resources for the most-significant risks. Considering fraud risks to which Medicare is most vulnerable, in light of the malicious intent of those who aim to exploit the programs, would help CMS to examine its current

---

[35] GAO, Results-Oriented Cultures: Implementation Steps to Assist Mergers and Organizational Transformations, GAO-03-669 (Washington, D.C.: July 2, 2003).

control activities and potentially design new ones with recognition of fraudulent behavior it aims to prevent. This focus on fraud is distinct from a broader view of program integrity and improper payments by considering the intentions and incentives of those who aim to deceive rather than well-intentioned providers who make mistakes. Also, continued growth of the program, such as growth of Medicare Part C, calls for consideration of preventive fraud control activities across the entire network of entities involved.

Furthermore, considering the large size and complexity of Medicare and the extensive stakeholder network involved in managing fraud in the program, a strategic approach to managing fraud risks within the programs is essential to ensure that a number of existing control activities and numerous stakeholder relationships and incentives are being aligned to produce desired results. Once developed, an antifraud strategy that is clearly articulated to various CMS stakeholders would help CMS to address fraud risks in a more coordinated and deliberate fashion.

Thinking strategically about existing control activities, resources, tools, and information systems could help CMS to leverage resources while continuing to integrate Medicare program-integrity efforts along functional lines. A strategic approach grounded in a comprehensive assessment of fraud risks could also help CMS to identify future enhancements for existing control activities, such as new preventive capabilities for its Fraud Prevention System (FPS) or additional fraud factors in provider enrollment and revalidation, such as provider risk-scoring, to stay in step with evolving fraud risks.

CMS Has Established Monitoring and Evaluation Mechanisms That Could Inform a Risk-Based Antifraud Strategy for Medicare

The *evaluate and adapt* component of the Fraud Risk Framework calls for federal managers to evaluate outcomes using a risk-based approach and adapt activities to improve fraud risk management. Furthermore, according to federal internal control standards, managers should establish and operate monitoring activities to monitor the internal control system and evaluate the results, which may be compared against an established baseline.[36] Ongoing monitoring and periodic evaluations provide assurances to managers that they are effectively preventing, detecting, and responding to potential fraud.

CMS has established monitoring and evaluation mechanisms for its program-integrity activities that it could incorporate into an antifraud strategy.

As described in the Fraud Risk Framework, agencies can gather information on the short-term or intermediate outcomes of some antifraud initiatives, which may be more readily measured. For example, CMS has developed some performance measures to provide a basis for monitoring its progress towards meeting the program-integrity goals set in the HHS Strategic Plan and Annual Performance Plan. Specifically, CMS measures whether it is meeting its goal of "increasing the percentage of Medicare FFS providers and suppliers identified as high risk that receive an administrative action."[37] CMS does not set specific antifraud goals for other parts of Medicare; other CMS performance measures relate to measuring or reducing improper payments in the various parts of Medicare.

CMS uses return-on-investment and savings estimates to measure the effectiveness of its Medicare program-integrity activities and FPS.[38] For example, CMS uses return-on-investment to measure the effectiveness of FPS[39] and, in response to a recommendation we made in 2012, CMS

---

[36] See GAO-14-704G.

[37] This performance metric refers to providers identified by FPS whose behavior is aberrant and potentially fraudulent. CMS can take a variety of administrative actions against those providers, from payment suspensions to revoking providers' billing privileges. CMS has met this goal from 2013 to 2015; the 2016 data were pending at the time of the writing of the December 2017 report.

[38] 38We previously found flaws with CMS's return-on-investment calculation and made two recommendations regarding the methodology. CMS has implemented both of the recommendations. See GAO, *Medicare Integrity Program: CMS Used Increased Funding for New Activities but Could Improve Measurement of Program Effectiveness*, GAO-11-592 (Washington, D.C.: July 29, 2011).

[39] HHS OIG has reviewed CMS's methodology and calculations and certified the use of adjusted savings, which in 2014 yielded the FPS return-on-investment of approximately 3 to 1.

developed outcome-based performance targets and milestones for FPS.[40] CMS has also conducted individual evaluations of its program-integrity activities, such as an interim evaluation of the prior-authorization demonstration for power mobility devices that began in 2012 and is currently implemented in 19 states.

Commensurate with greater maturity of control activities in Medicare FFS compared to other parts of Medicare and Medicaid, monitoring and evaluation activities for Medicare Parts C and D and Medicaid are more limited. For example, CMS calculates savings for its program-integrity activities in Medicare Parts C and D, but not a full return-on-investment. CMS officials told us that calculating costs for specific activities is challenging because of overlapping activities among contractors. CMS officials said they continue to refine methods and develop new savings estimates for additional program-integrity activities.

According to the Fraud Risk Framework, effective managers develop a strategy and evaluate outcomes using a risk-based approach. In developing an effective strategy and antifraud activities, managers consider the benefits and costs of control activities. Ongoing monitoring and periodic evaluations provide reasonable assurance to managers that they are effectively preventing, detecting, and responding to potential fraud. Monitoring and evaluation activities can also support managers' decisions about allocating resources, and help them to demonstrate their continued commitment to effectively managing fraud risks.

As CMS takes steps to develop an antifraud strategy, it could include plans for refining and building on existing methods such as return-on-investment or savings measures, and setting appropriate targets to evaluate the effectiveness of all of CMS's antifraud efforts. Such a strategy would help CMS to efficiently allocate program-integrity resources and to ensure that the agency is effectively preventing, detecting, and responding to potential fraud. For example, while doing so would involve challenges, CMS's strategy could detail plans to advance efforts to measure a

---

[40] GAO, Medicare Fraud Prevention: CMS Has Implemented a Predictive Analytics System, but Needs to Define Measures to Determine Its Effectiveness, GAO-13-104 (Washington, D.C.: Oct. 15, 2012).

potential fraud rate through baseline and periodic measures. Fraud-rate measurement efforts could also inform risk assessment activities, identify currently unknown fraud risks, align resources to priority risks, and develop effective outcome metrics for antifraud controls. Such a strategy would also help CMS ensure that it has effective performance measures in place to assess its antifraud efforts beyond those related to providers in Medicare FFS, and establish appropriate targets to measure the agency's progress in addressing fraud risks.

In our December 2017 report we recommended that the Administrator of CMS should, using the results of the fraud risk assessments for Medicare, create, document, implement, and communicate an antifraud strategy that is aligned with and responsive to regularly assessed fraud risks. This strategy should include an approach for monitoring and evaluation. In its March 2018 letter to GAO, HHS stated that it is currently evaluating its options with regards to implementing this recommendation. As of July 2018, the recommendation remains open.

Chairman Jenkins and Ranking Member Lewis, this concludes my prepared statement. I look forward to the subcommittee's questions.

GAO Contacts and Staff Acknowledgments

If you or your staff have any questions concerning this testimony, please contact Seto J. Bagdoyan, who may be reached at (202) 512-6722 or bagdoyans@gao.gov. Contact points for our Offices of Congressional Relations and Public Affairs may be found on the last page of this statement. Other individuals who made key contributions to this testimony include Tonita Gillich (Assistant Director), Irina Carnevale (Analyst-in-Charge), Colin Fallon, Scott Hiromoto, and Maria McMullen.

INDEX

A

abuse, 7, 8, 75, 86, 113, 116, 121, 122, 124, 139, 140, 147, 149, 154, 155, 158, 159, 160, 161, 164, 170
adjustment, 54, 125, 134
Affordable Care Act (ACA), ix, 4, 9, 10, 11, 18, 21, 24, 34, 35, 167
age, ix, 2, 17, 20, 25, 45, 48
agencies, 20, 40, 48, 67, 68, 92, 95, 121, 123, 124, 127, 130, 146, 147, 148, 150, 155, 156, 160, 167, 171, 173
aging population, 62
appropriations, vii, ix, 18, 38, 40, 44, 64
assessment, 132, 147, 155, 163, 164, 166, 167, 168, 172
assets, 5, 6, 9, 11, 13, 14, 23, 27, 31, 32, 38, 40, 41, 52, 64
atmospheric pressure, 69
audit(s), 72, 113, 116, 123, 150, 166

B

balance sheet, 5, 23
bankruptcy, 13, 23
base year, 10
behaviors, 165

beneficiaries, viii, ix, 1, 2, 3, 5, 13, 17, 19, 20, 22, 23, 24, 28, 29, 38, 39, 45, 46, 47, 48, 51, 54, 55, 56, 73, 75, 76, 78, 87, 89, 90, 111, 112, 114, 115, 120, 132, 141, 149, 151, 152, 160, 168
benefits, ix, x, 3, 4, 5, 9, 11, 13, 14, 15, 18, 19, 21, 22, 23, 25, 26, 33, 46, 47, 50, 52, 55, 56, 57, 66, 67, 70, 71, 88, 92, 96, 151, 174
bonuses, 34
budgetary resources, 14, 38, 49, 64

C

cash, 5, 6, 22
cash flow, 6
Centers for Medicare and Medicaid Services (CMS), ix, 17
CFR, 56, 85
challenges, x, 66, 67, 70, 71, 89, 133, 137, 139, 154, 174
chemotherapy, 74
claims data, x, 117, 118, 119, 121, 131, 132, 138, 140, 141
classification, 20, 48
clinical judgment, 129
coding, 111, 115

cognitive impairment, 89
collaboration, x, 118, 119, 123, 130, 140, 160, 168
communication, 159, 168
competition, 171
complexity, viii, xi, 3, 28, 69, 120, 145, 149, 154, 166, 167, 172
compliance, 66, 68, 71, 83, 160, 162, 165
computing, 57
conference, 170
configuration, 101
Congress, viii, ix, x, 2, 3, 6, 8, 13, 18, 20, 27, 37, 38, 39, 41, 44, 45, 54, 58, 59, 60, 61, 62, 63, 118, 122, 125, 134, 148, 150, 157, 170
Congressional Budget Office, 14, 46, 61, 62, 149, 152
conspiracy, 148
consumer price index, 3, 21
cost, ix, 3, 18, 20, 24, 25, 29, 31, 48, 51, 53, 54, 55, 120, 151, 154
cost saving, 154
covering, 26, 31, 105
CPI, 21, 120, 124, 125, 130, 137, 147, 158, 159, 163, 164, 165, 167, 168, 170
creditors, 13, 23

D

data analysis, 124, 127, 133, 160, 168
deficiency, 101
deficit, ix, 5, 18, 27, 30, 32, 34, 42, 44, 45, 63
demonstrations, viii, x, 66, 68, 69, 70, 71, 73, 78, 79, 80, 81, 83, 84, 85, 91, 93, 94, 96, 97, 111, 112, 114, 115, 116
denial, 128, 134
Department of Defense, 41, 58, 130
Department of Health and Human Services, 48, 66, 68, 69, 98, 110, 111, 114, 119, 120, 121, 128, 136, 146, 148, 149

Department of Justice, 48, 128, 130, 148, 149, 165
Department of the Treasury, 3, 20, 21
detection, 166, 169
diabetes, 33, 159
dialysis, 74
disability, 20, 48
distribution, 97, 142
District of Columbia, 74, 82, 106, 107, 108, 109
doctors, 20, 48
drugs, 33

E

earnings, 2, 4, 16, 19, 21, 46
economic downturn, 28
economic growth, 7, 8
education, 42, 49, 54, 80, 86, 87, 160
educational materials, 160
emergency, 56, 69, 70, 71, 73, 74, 75, 78, 79, 80, 81, 82, 84, 86, 89, 94, 95
employees, 4, 146, 157, 160, 161, 165, 170
employers, vii, viii, 1, 4, 5, 21, 22, 46, 57
employment, 4
end-stage renal disease, 20, 46, 48, 69, 120, 151
enforcement, 37, 38, 39, 41, 45, 48, 135, 148, 155, 160, 168
enrollment, 3, 8, 48, 85, 86, 159, 162, 163, 167, 169, 170, 172
environment, 168
equipment, ix, 2, 17, 19, 20, 46, 48, 67, 68, 69, 73, 77, 85, 86, 87, 90, 95, 98, 120, 129, 149
evidence, 72, 118, 123, 127, 128, 132, 136, 140, 150
execution, 40
Executive Order, 158
expenditures, vii, ix, x, 3, 6, 8, 9, 10, 11, 13, 14, 18, 24, 25, 26, 27, 28, 29, 30, 32, 33,

34, 35, 66, 69, 70, 71, 73, 74, 75, 80, 81, 83, 84, 85, 86, 87, 96, 105, 111, 112, 115, 149, 169

F

false positive, 139
Federal Bureau of Investigation, 48, 168
federal government, 13, 23, 40, 53, 63, 69, 72, 155
federal insurance, ix, 2, 17
federal law, 63
Federal Register, 72
fee-for-service, x, 117, 130
financial data, 14
financial incentives, 90
financial resources, 29
financial soundness, 30
fiscal year, vii, x, xi, 38, 40, 45, 51, 52, 59, 69, 97, 118, 119, 120, 122, 123, 133, 134, 135, 137, 145, 148, 149, 151, 154, 168
flexibility, 5, 22, 133
fluid, 104
FPS (Fraud Prevention System), v, x, 117, 118, 119, 120, 121, 122, 123, 124, 125, 127, 130, 131, 132, 133, 134, 135, 136, 137, 162, 172, 173
fraud, viii, x, xi, 7, 42, 48, 58, 73, 74, 75, 76, 86, 98, 111, 113, 115, 116, 117, 118, 119, 121, 122, 123, 124, 125, 126, 127, 128, 130, 131, 132, 133, 135, 136, 137, 138, 139, 140, 141, 145, 146, 147, 148, 149, 150, 154, 155, 156, 157, 158, 159, 160, 161, 162, 163, 164, 165, 166, 167, 168, 169, 170, 171, 172, 174, 175
friction, 101, 102, 103, 104
funding, 4, 13, 24, 27, 31, 40, 41, 42, 44, 49, 52, 58, 59, 60, 61, 62
funds, vii, viii, 2, 3, 4, 13, 14, 20, 21, 23, 27, 38, 40, 41, 48, 50, 51, 52, 58, 59, 63, 124

G

GAO, x, xi, 40, 41, 52, 64, 65, 66, 67, 69, 72, 76, 77, 79, 80, 81, 82, 84, 85, 86, 87, 88, 90, 92, 95, 98, 105, 106, 107, 108, 109, 110, 111, 112, 113, 114, 115, 116, 117, 118, 119, 120, 124, 126, 127, 128, 129, 132, 133, 134, 135, 136, 139, 142, 144, 145, 146, 147, 148, 149, 150, 151, 152, 154, 155, 156, 158, 159, 161, 162, 163, 164, 166, 167, 169, 171, 173, 174, 175
GDP, 11, 28, 29, 30, 32, 33, 34, 35, 149, 152
gel, 103
genetic testing, 139
government securities, 5, 22
government spending, 5, 22, 41, 58
greed, 146
growth, viii, ix, 2, 3, 6, 9, 10, 11, 17, 18, 27, 28, 29, 33, 56, 57, 172
growth rate, 33, 57
guidance, 53, 89, 146, 148, 155, 156
guidelines, 156

H

Hatch, Orrin, 68
healing, 75
health, vii, viii, ix, x, 1, 2, 3, 8, 10, 13, 17, 18, 20, 28, 29, 38, 39, 42, 45, 46, 47, 48, 55, 58, 62, 66, 68, 69, 70, 72, 73, 75, 77, 78, 80, 82, 84, 85, 86, 90, 91, 94, 97, 111, 112, 114, 115, 116, 117, 118, 119, 120, 121, 122, 123, 130, 133, 136, 138, 139, 141, 145, 147, 148, 149, 151, 154, 155, 160, 162, 165, 168, 171
Health and Human Services, 97, 142
health care, ix, x, 2, 3, 8, 10, 13, 17, 28, 29, 38, 39, 42, 45, 46, 47, 48, 58, 62, 66, 68,

69, 85, 90, 111, 114, 117, 118, 119, 121, 122, 123, 130, 136, 138
health care costs, 8, 13, 62
health care programs, 85, 130
health care system, ix, 18
health expenditure, 28
health information, 141
health insurance, vii, viii, ix, 1, 2, 17, 47, 69, 120, 151
health services, ix, 17, 18, 28, 46, 70, 73, 75, 77, 78, 80, 82, 84, 86, 91, 94, 97, 111, 112, 115, 116, 120
Healthcare Fraud Prevention Partnership (HFPP), x, 117, 118, 119, 120, 121, 122, 123, 130, 138, 139, 140, 141, 160
health-care sector, vii, x, 145, 149
height, 101, 105
hepatitis, 33
HHS, 46, 48, 54, 56, 57, 68, 69, 76, 95, 97, 111, 112, 113, 114, 115, 116, 120, 121, 125, 128, 130, 136, 142, 148, 149, 161, 168, 169, 173, 175
HI Trust Fund, vii, viii, 1, 2, 3, 4, 5, 6, 8, 9, 10, 11, 12, 13, 14, 21, 22, 23, 26, 27, 31, 32, 61
hip joint, 101, 102, 103
historical data, 29
hospice, 2, 18, 19, 20, 46, 47, 48, 55, 120
Hospital Insurance, vii, viii, 1, 3, 5, 7, 10, 11, 12, 14, 15, 19, 20, 21, 22, 25, 28, 46
House of Representatives, 18, 142, 143, 144, 145
hyperbaric oxygen therapy, 69, 71, 73, 75, 78, 80, 81, 82, 84, 89, 94, 111, 115

I

improvements, 6, 8, 76, 94
income, 4, 5, 9, 10, 11, 12, 13, 14, 15, 21, 22, 23, 24, 25, 26, 27, 30, 31, 32, 42, 51, 57

income tax, 4, 11, 14, 21, 30
individuals, ix, 2, 17, 24, 69, 85, 120, 130, 148, 151, 175
inflation, 3, 76, 98
information sharing, 119, 140, 160, 168, 171
information technology, x, 42, 49, 118, 119, 120, 122
infrastructure, 42, 49
integrity, x, 48, 58, 67, 69, 71, 85, 86, 96, 111, 114, 117, 118, 121, 122, 124, 126, 127, 128, 132, 133, 135, 136, 147, 155, 157, 158, 160, 170, 171, 172, 173, 174
interface, 99
intermediaries, 91
internal controls, 72, 156, 161
investment, 147, 173, 174

J

joints, 101, 104
jurisdiction, 122, 126, 133

L

law enforcement, 127, 128, 130, 134, 135
laws, 6, 37, 38, 39, 40, 64
leadership, 158, 170
legislation, ix, 6, 10, 11, 18, 32, 33, 42, 44, 45, 63
life expectancy, 3, 21
light, 104, 105, 165, 171
liquidate, 63
logistics, 140
Louisiana, 74, 82, 106

M

majority, 161

management, xi, 59, 72, 104, 132, 146, 150, 155, 157, 158, 159, 163, 169
market share, 72
marketplace, 167
Maryland, 74, 82, 106, 107
Medicaid, viii, ix, xi, 8, 11, 17, 19, 20, 24, 40, 47, 48, 51, 53, 54, 56, 57, 61, 66, 68, 69, 77, 79, 80, 82, 84, 85, 98, 106, 107, 108, 109, 112, 115, 118, 120, 121, 122, 126, 130, 134, 146, 148, 149, 150, 151, 159, 160, 161, 168, 169, 170, 171, 174
medical care, 129
medical practices, ix, 18, 121
medical services, ix, 2, 3, 17, 19, 46, 147
Medicare,
    Advantage, vii, viii, 1, 2, 7, 9, 19, 32, 33, 47, 55, 56, 57, 61, 72, 123, 151, 165, 166
    Spending, vii, ix, 6, 10, 13, 14, 18, 25, 28, 31, 38, 46
    Trustees Report, vii, viii, 2, 3, 6, 7, 8, 9, 10, 12, 16, 25, 28, 33
medicine, ix, 17
membership, 123, 130
methodology, 10, 85, 150, 173
metropolitan areas, 87
military, 43, 44
miniature, 104
MIP, 42, 43, 46, 48, 49, 58
missions, 168
Missouri, 74, 76, 82, 106
models, 34, 70, 111, 114, 115, 124, 169
moratorium, 86

N

negotiating, 140
networking, 140
nursing, 2, 10, 18, 20, 46, 48, 120, 149
nursing care, 18, 46

O

Office of Management and Budget (OMB), 41, 154, 156
Office of the Inspector General, 95
officials, x, xi, 66, 67, 71, 72, 74, 78, 80, 83, 85, 86, 88, 89, 90, 91, 92, 93, 94, 95, 96, 118, 119, 122, 123, 131, 132, 133, 136, 137, 138, 139, 141, 146, 155, 158, 159, 163, 164, 165, 167, 168, 170, 171, 174
opportunities, 68, 70, 95, 96, 97, 112, 116, 154, 165
organizational culture, 157, 158
outpatient, vii, viii, 1, 2, 9, 14, 19, 20, 46, 47, 48, 69, 120, 125, 129, 151
outpatient prescription drug benefit, vii, viii, 1, 19, 47
outreach, 42, 49, 53, 54, 86, 87, 160
overlay, 99
oxygen, 69, 70, 75, 94, 95

P

Part A, vii, viii, 1, 2, 3, 4, 5, 7, 9, 10, 11, 12, 13, 14, 18, 19, 20, 21, 22, 23, 25, 26, 27, 29, 30, 32, 46, 47, 51, 53, 61, 69, 120, 129, 151
Part B, vii, viii, 1, 2, 3, 19, 22, 23, 24, 25, 26, 29, 30, 32, 33, 43, 46, 47, 49, 51, 53, 55, 61, 69, 120, 129, 151
Part C, vii, viii, 1, 2, 3, 6, 7, 8, 19, 20, 25, 47, 55, 56, 57, 60, 61, 72, 151, 165, 166, 168, 172
Part D, vii, viii, 1, 2, 3, 9, 19, 23, 24, 25, 26, 29, 30, 32, 33, 42, 47, 51, 55, 56, 57, 151
participants, x, 118, 119, 123, 130, 138, 139, 140, 141
Patient Protection and Affordable Care Act (ACA), 4, 21, 24

payroll, vii, viii, 1, 2, 3, 4, 5, 6, 7, 8, 9, 10, 11, 14, 18, 21, 22, 23, 26, 30, 31, 32, 34, 46
payroll taxes, vii, viii, 1, 2, 3, 4, 5, 7, 9, 11, 14, 18, 21, 22, 23, 26, 30, 31, 32, 34, 46
physicians, ix, 17, 18, 34, 53, 67, 78, 89, 91, 121, 136, 149
plantar flexion, 105
population, 28, 149
prescription drugs, 24, 139
present value, 30, 31
prevention, 124, 159, 161, 166, 168, 169, 170
primary function, 124
prior authorization, viii, ix, x, 65, 66, 67, 68, 69, 70, 71, 72, 73, 74, 75, 76, 77, 78, 79, 80, 81, 83, 85, 87, 88, 89, 90, 91, 92, 93, 94, 95, 96, 97, 98, 105, 111, 112, 113, 114, 115, 116, 162
private health plans, viii, 1, 55, 149
private sector, 20
profit margin, 56
program administration, 25
project, 10, 13, 27, 28, 30
prosthesis, 101, 104, 105

Q

quality improvement, 42, 49

R

real wage, 10
recession, 9
recognition, 172
recommendations, 54, 66, 96, 97, 112, 116, 146, 166, 173
reconciliation, 6
recovery, 9, 166
regulations, 56
rehabilitation, 20, 48

reimburse, 20, 48, 56
reinsurance, 42, 51, 57
reliability, 122, 123
reputation, 165
requirement, 133
requirements, ix, 18, 56, 65, 77, 78, 85, 87, 89, 90, 91, 92, 95, 119, 121, 125, 129, 133, 148, 159, 160
resources, 5, 38, 40, 42, 49, 51, 59, 60, 62, 63, 64, 131, 137, 167, 171, 172, 174
response, 89, 97, 105, 125, 135, 158, 166, 167, 173
restitution, 148
revenue, 3, 14, 23, 24, 25, 26, 27, 30, 31, 32, 42, 56
risk, 20, 48, 55, 57, 69, 72, 85, 113, 116, 119, 120, 125, 127, 133, 136, 139, 146, 147, 149, 151, 154, 155, 156, 157, 159, 161, 162, 163, 164, 165, 166, 167, 168, 169, 170, 171, 172, 173, 174, 175
risk assessment, 72, 146, 147, 157, 162, 163, 164, 165, 166, 167, 168, 169, 170, 171, 175
risk factors, 20, 48, 165
risk management, 147, 150, 156, 157, 161, 169, 172
risk profile, 147, 162, 163, 164, 166, 169
rules, vii, ix, 32, 37, 38, 39, 40, 41, 42, 45, 49, 51, 52, 54, 65, 66, 68, 72, 77, 78, 96, 111, 115, 119, 129, 135, 136, 139, 162

S

savings, x, 8, 41, 50, 51, 55, 62, 63, 66, 67, 68, 70, 81, 83, 84, 95, 96, 118, 122, 123, 125, 134, 135, 137, 147, 173, 174
scope, 76, 98, 148, 150, 154, 167
securities, 4, 5, 12, 21, 22, 23
security, 41
self-employed, 4
Senate, 39, 65, 68

Index 183

services, viii, ix, x, 1, 2, 3, 5, 9, 10, 12, 13, 17, 18, 19, 20, 22, 27, 28, 29, 33, 38, 39, 45, 46, 47, 48, 51, 53, 54, 55, 56, 66, 69, 70, 71, 72, 73, 74, 75, 77, 79, 80, 81, 82, 84, 85, 86, 88, 89, 90, 91, 94, 95, 96, 97, 105, 111, 112, 113, 115, 116, 119, 120, 121, 125, 129, 131, 132, 136, 137, 138, 139, 140, 147, 148, 151, 159, 162
shortfall, vii, viii, 2, 3, 13, 24, 27, 31
skin, 89
Social Security, 2, 3, 4, 5, 6, 11, 12, 13, 14, 15, 19, 21, 24, 27, 30, 33, 40, 41, 43, 45, 46, 49, 50, 53, 58, 64, 73, 74, 75, 76, 111, 115
spending, vii, viii, ix, 2, 5, 6, 8, 10, 13, 14, 18, 19, 23, 25, 26, 27, 28, 31, 32, 33, 37, 38, 39, 40, 41, 42, 43, 44, 45, 46, 47, 49, 50, 52, 56, 58, 59, 61, 63, 64, 75, 152
staff members, 142
stakeholder groups, 147, 160
stakeholders, xi, 71, 96, 146, 147, 155, 158, 159, 160, 161, 163, 168, 169, 170, 171, 172
statistics, 149
statutory authority, 13, 73, 97, 113, 116
structural changes, 28
subsidy, 24, 57
Supplemental Nutrition Assistance Program, 64
Supplementary Medical Insurance, vii, viii, 1, 3, 5, 11, 12, 15, 19, 20, 22, 23, 25, 46
supplier(s), x, 17, 20, 48, 54, 66, 67, 68, 71, 78, 80, 83, 85, 86, 87, 88, 89, 90, 91, 92, 93, 96, 112, 115, 149, 159
surplus, 5, 14, 26, 27
susceptibility, 69, 120, 149
suspensions, 128, 135, 173

T

target, 85, 119, 136, 147, 162, 171

tax rates, 6
taxation, 14, 15, 33
taxes, vii, viii, 1, 2, 3, 4, 5, 7, 9, 11, 14, 18, 21, 22, 23, 26, 30, 31, 32, 34, 46
taxpayers, 13
technical comments, 97, 119, 142
technology, ix, 18, 76
therapy, 33, 69, 75, 99
threats, 165
time periods, 70
titanium, 104, 105
Title I, 44
Title IV, 44
tracks, 119
training, 146, 147, 157, 160, 161
transfer of money, 21
transfer payments, 24, 26
transparency, 170
transport, 70, 86, 111, 115
transportation, 74
Treasury, 5, 6, 12, 21, 22, 23
trust fund, vii, viii, xi, 1, 2, 3, 4, 5, 6, 7, 8, 9, 10, 11, 12, 13, 14, 15, 19, 20, 21, 22, 23, 24, 25, 26, 27, 31, 32, 46, 47, 61, 145, 149

U

U.S. economy, vii, x, 29, 145, 149
U.S. Treasury, 4, 21
urine, 139

V

vulnerability, 119, 136, 161

W

wage increases, 3, 21
wages, 4, 11, 21, 32

Washington, 68, 69, 72, 74, 82, 85, 86, 87, 88, 90, 95, 106, 110, 114, 120, 124, 132, 133, 136, 148, 149, 150, 154, 155, 156, 159, 162, 167, 171, 173, 174

waste, 42, 48, 58, 86, 113, 116, 121, 122, 124, 139, 147, 149, 154, 155, 158, 159, 160, 161, 164, 170

workers, vii, viii, 1, 3, 4, 5, 10, 16, 21, 22, 46, 57

workforce, 3, 21, 147, 161

workload, 132, 133

Translational Research: Recent Progress and Future Directions

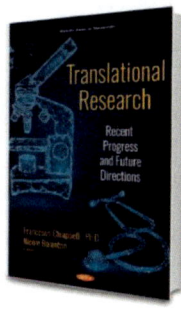

Editors: Francesco Chiappelli, Ph.D. (University of California at Los Angeles School of Dentistry, California State University, Northridge, CA, USA); Nicole Balenton (UCLA Center for the Health Sciences School of Nursing, Los Angeles, CA USA)

Series: Health Care in Transition

Book Description: The chapters in this book highlight the transfer of basic science discovered and cutting-edge developments into clinical applications.

Hardcover ISBN: 978-1-53614-598-4
Retail Price: $230

Fundamentals of Leadership for Healthcare Professionals

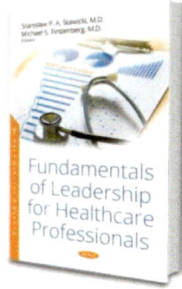

Editors: Stanislaw P. A. Stawicki, M.D. (Department of Research and Innovation, St Luke's University Health Network, Bethlehem, Pennsylvania, US); Michael S. Firstenberg, M.D. (Department of Surgery (Cardiothoracic), The Medical Center of Aurora, Aurora, Colorado, US)

Series: Health Care in Transition

Book Description: Each chapter in this text explores different aspects of healthcare leadership, provides valuable insights into how effective leadership functions, and offers practical perspectives on implementations of theory into practice.

Hardcover ISBN: 978-1-53613-620-3
Retail Price: $195

Pandemics: Evolutionary Engineering of Consciousness and Health

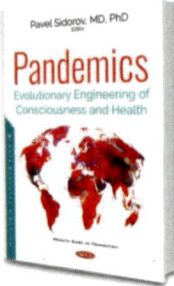

Editor: Pavel I. Sidorov, M.D., Ph.D. (Institute of Mental Medicine, Northern State Medical University, Arkhangelsk, Russia)

Series: Health Care in Transition

Book Description: In this book, the authors have analyzed new epigenetic and etiopathogenesis mechanisms, pathomorphosis and pathokinetics of clinical manifestations of classic and new pandemics, from influenza to mental illnesses.

Softcover ISBN: 978-1-53614-274-7
Retail Price: $95